WHAT'S IN YOUR FOOD?

Bill Statham

WHAT'S IN YOUR FOOD?

The Truth About Food Additives From Aspartame to Xanthan Gum

Bill Statham

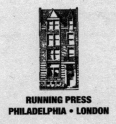

RUNNING PRESS
PHILADELPHIA • LONDON

First published in Australia and New Zealand as *The Chemical Maze*, by possibility.com in 2002

First UK edition published as *The Chemical Maze Shopping Companion*, by Summersdale Publishers Ltd. in 2006

© 2007 (North American Edition) by Bill Statham

9 8 7 6 5 4 3 2 1

Digit on the right indicates the number of this printing

Library of Congress Control Number: 2006934558

ISBN-13: 978-0-7624-2963-9

ISBN-10: 0-7624-2963-1

Cover design by Bill Jones

Interior design by Bill Jones and Scribe, Inc. (www.scribenet.com)

Typography: Scribe, Inc. (www.scribenet.com)

This book may be ordered by mail from the publisher. Please include $2.50 for postage and handling.

But try your bookstore first!

Running Press Book Publishers

2300 Chestnut Street

Philadelphia, PA 19103

Visit us on the web!

www.runningpress.com

TABLE OF CONTENTS

FOREWORD

Both new and experienced "safe consumers" will benefit from Bill Statham's research and guidance in *What's in Your Food?*

Do not be deceived by its miniature size—this little handbook could create big changes in the way you look at food and personal care forever. If you take Bill's advice to heart, no longer will you be able to participate in mindless shopping expeditions. Ignorance may once have been bliss, but now it spells danger in our mass-manufactured, profit-driven, long shelf-life, chemical-romanced society.

After spending many years researching the toxic ingredients in skin and personal care, and successfully avoiding all of them in the products I create, I am happy to recommend Bill Statham's *What's in Your Food?* as an excellent reference guide to anyone questioning the safety of those strange-sounding "naturally derived" ingredients in their skin and personal care.

Moreover, as a long-term Certified Organic consumer, I truly hope you put your money where your health is, and "Go Organic"!

Narelle Chenery
Director of Research and Development, Miessence

HOW TO USE YOUR GUIDE

The reference part of this book is divided into two sections.

Section One provides an alphabetical list of **food additives** that may be found in **food products**. Section Two provides an alphabetical list of **ingredients** that may be found in **cosmetics and personal care products.** Some ingredients are also used as food additives, therefore to avoid unnecessary repetition, they may be found in Section One. Examples are beeswax, bentonite, candelilla wax, and glycerin.

A glossary at the end explains certain terms and abbreviations you may be unfamiliar with (i.e.—CNS, surfactant).

A face code shows just how user-friendly each additive/ingredient is, from *safe and/or beneficial* through to *hazardous*.

☺☺	2 happy faces = safe and/or beneficial
☺	1 happy face = safe for most people
☺?	1 quizzical face = caution advised
☹	1 sad face = best avoided
☹☹	2 sad faces = hazardous

A system of color coding: dark for "to be avoided," gray for "wait/caution," and white for "proceed safely" makes reading the tables even simpler.

Note: The evaluation given is the opinion of the author at the time of writing based on available researched information. This information was referenced from several sources, including but not limited to: Material Safety Data Sheets, animal studies, medical, and scientific laboratory reports.

The codes shown are only a general guide, as individuals react differently to chemical exposures. The type and severity of reaction will depend on many factors. A few of these are: the health of the person, the amounts to which they are exposed and the period of exposure, the environment in which the person lives/works, and the person's age and gender. However, it is recommended that only those products containing additives and ingredients that are *safe and/or beneficial* or *safe for most people* as indicated by the happy faces be chosen.

The tables also show some of the benefits of the additive/ingredient and/or some of the detrimental effects, symptoms and illnesses it has the potential to either cause or exacerbate, and some of the environmental effects that may occur.

In most cases the origin of each additive/ingredient is also given, including whether it may be of animal origin or a product of genetic engineering (GE).

Where certain specific medical disorders including cancer, diabetes, tumors, and others are mentioned, only limited reference is made as to whether occurrence was in animals or humans. Also, usually no reference is made to the amounts or concentration of chemicals involved, types of exposure or time periods involved. This information is far beyond the scope of this book, and the reader is directed to the bibliography if they wish to find out more information. The tables also list a few relevant, common consumer products that may contain that particular additive/ingredient, and some other possible uses for it.

Beyond the tables, there is also a section on genetic engineering and, for those who want more information than can be included in a book of this size, a list of useful Internet resources.

DISCLAIMER

Every effort has been made to ensure that the information in this book is accurate and current at the time of publication. The book does not claim to include all information about all chemicals used in foods, cosmetics and personal care products. The author and the publisher disclaim liability for any misuse or misunderstanding of any information contained herein and disclaims liability for all loss, damage or injury, be it health, financial or otherwise, suffered by any individual or group acting upon or relying on information contained herein. The information given should not be construed as medical advice and a qualified health practitioner should be consulted in all cases of ill health.

INTRODUCTION

"Like the constant dripping of water that wears away the hardest stone, (the) birth to death contact with dangerous chemicals may in the end prove disastrous. Each of these recurrent exposures, no matter how slight, culminates in the progressive build-up of chemicals in our bodies and so to cumulative poisoning... Lulled by the soft sell and the hidden persuader; the average citizen is seldom aware of the deadly materials with which he is surrounding himself; indeed, he may not realize he is using them at all."

Rachel Carson, *Silent Spring* (1962)

The idea for this book was born out of a need to understand how some chemicals that are a part of our everyday lives may also play a part in ill health. As a homeopathic practitioner, I often wondered why some of my patients would regain their health under treatment only to relapse later. It was only after some research that I made the connection between what my patients were eating—not just the types of foods, but also often more significantly the chemical food additives that they contained—and their health problems. I also investigated whether there was a possibility that the products they used on their bodies every day, personal care and cosmetic products, could also have a detrimental effect on their health.

What I discovered during my research amazed and often shocked me. I discovered that a significant number of chemicals added to foods and cosmetics could cause or exacerbate health problems such as asthma, dermatitis, hives, migraines, hay fever, gastric upsets, behavioral problems, hyperactivity, learning difficulties, and many others. Some of these chemicals are found to be toxic to body organs and systems like the liver, kidneys, heart, thymus, brain, immune, nervous, hormonal, and endocrine systems. Even more disturbing was the fact that some chemicals permitted in foods, personal care products and cosmetics could also cause damage to DNA, birth defects, genetic mutations, and cancer. I began to tell my patients of my discoveries and encouraged them to eliminate, as much as possible, the chemicals that were found to have detrimental effects on health. As I had expected, the health of my patients improved dramatically and often surprised even the patients themselves.

An interesting side effect happened as well. Those patients who enrolled their families and friends into this new lifestyle by eliminating harmful chemicals were reporting that the health and well being of these people was also improving, sometimes dramatically so.

I came to the decision that perhaps I should write a booklet so that many people could benefit from this knowledge. I had envisioned a credit card sized guide that would fit in the wallet. It wasn't long into the research that I realized that the information would overflow such a small format. I plowed on with my research and after another twelve months felt I had enough information to publish a small shopping guide.

The first edition of this book was self-published—as *The Chemical Maze*—in Australia in April 2001. Five years later, over 50,000 copies had been sold, mostly in Australia and New Zealand. Since the first edition found its way into homes and shopping bags, I have received many letters and emails from people thanking me for producing a user-friendly guide to the vast array of additives and ingredients in our foods, cosmetics and personal care products, and telling me how their health and that of their children has improved after using the book to eliminate harmful chemicals from their lives. I am often touched and inspired by the stories they tell, like the following from Debra in Sydney:

"I would like to share with you a miracle with my youngest son Jack. By eliminating harmful chemicals from our house and processed food, my son's behavior has become much calmer. The main difference that we welcomed was related to Jack's typical ADHD symptoms (not that I ever put him in that

box). This is the first time that anything had actually made a huge difference for him. His memory is getting better each day and he is able to learn more easily than before. His Rudolf Steiner schoolteacher is amazed at the dramatic difference."

This book provides information on almost 600 food additives and over 450 of the most common ingredients found in cosmetics and personal care products. Manufacturers can choose from well in excess of *10,000* substances, of which more than 1000 are know to have harmful effects. It's impossible to list all of them in a user-friendly guide, so this book contains those you are most likely to encounter regularly.

A frightening number of the chemicals manufacturers use have never been adequately tested for long-term effects on human health. In addition, there are ingredients in use here that some other countries have banned.

Looking on the positive side, there are an increasing number of companies producing foods and cosmetic products without harmful additives and synthetic chemicals. So we do have choices, and, with a little bit of guidance and a determination to act, we can avoid the nasty ones and lead healthier lives. The price of ignorance and apathy can be very high indeed. We do not have to pay that price.

Our existence on this planet may well depend on the decisions we make and the actions we take.

Now is the time to act!

SECTION 1
FOOD ADDITIVES

Names	Function	Code	
Acacia gum (gum arabic; from *Acacia senegal*; on the NIH HSDB)	Thickener Emulsifier	☺?	
Acesulfame-potassium (synthetic chemical)	Artificial sweetener Flavor enhancer	☹	
Acetal (derived from acetaldehyde)	Flavoring Solvent	☹	
Acetaldehyde (ethanal; on the NIH HSDB)	Solvent Intermediate	☹☹	
Acetate (salt of acetic acid)	Flavoring	☺	
Acetic acid (occurs naturally in a variety of fruits and plants; on the NIH HSDB)	Acidifier Preservative Solvent	☹	

Potential Effects	Possible Food Use	Other Uses
Low oral toxicity; asthma; skin rash; hives; hay fever	Candy, soft drinks, chewing gum, jelly, glazes	Mascara, body wash, medicines, hair products
Caused lung tumors, breast tumors, respiratory disease, leukemia and cancer in animal studies	Tabletop sweeteners, low-calorie foods, chewing gum, beverages	Oral care products, toothpaste for dogs
Respiratory depression; cardiovascular collapse; CNS depression; high blood pressure	Artificial fruit flavoring in processed foods like beverages, ice cream, candy, chewing gum	Synthetic perfume, hypnotic in medicine
Skin & mucous membrane irritation; kidney, respiratory and neurotoxicity; liver damage; CNS depression; suspected teratogen; recognized carcinogen; toxic to aquatic organisms	Artificial flavoring in processed foods	Fragrance in cosmetics, perfume manufacture, silvering mirrors, synthetic rubber
Believed safe in food use at low levels; large quantities may cause stomach upset	Processed foods like beverages, ice cream, candy, baked goods	Perfumery
Cardiovascular, respiratory, gastrointestinal, liver and skin toxicity; hives; itching; skin irritation; toxic to aquatic organisms	Processed cheese, cheese spread, canned asparagus, processed meats	Hand lotion, hair dye, animal feeds, cigarettes

Names	Function	Code	
Acetoin (acetyl methyl carbinol; synthetic)	Flavoring Carrier	☺	
Acetone (by fermentation or oxidation; on the NIH HSDB)	Carrier or extraction solvent	☹	
Acetone peroxide (derived from acetone)	Maturing agent Bleaching agent	☺?	
Acetophenone (acetyl benzene; synthetic; may be from coal tar)	Flavoring	☺?	
Acetylated mono and diglycerides (synthetic; may be GE)	Emulsifier Release agent Glazing agent	☺☺	
Acetylated tartaric acid esters of mono-and diglycerides (synthetic; may be of ANIMAL origin; may be GE)	Emulsifier Thickener Stabilizer	☺	
Aconitic acid (mostly synthetic by dehydration of citric acid with sulfuric acid)	Flavoring	☺☺	

Potential Effects	Possible Food Use	Other Uses
Believed safe in food use; may cause skin irritation; moderately toxic if injected	Processed foods like beverages, ice cream, candy, baked goods	Perfumery
Cardiovascular, kidney, gastrointestinal, respiratory, liver, skin and neurotoxicity	Spice extraction, marking inks for eggs and meat	Nail polish, nail polish remover, shoe polish
Under investigation by the FDA for mutagenic, teratogenic, sub-acute and reproductive effects	Bleaching flour and dough, bakery products	Illicit explosive devices
Toxic by ingestion; skin toxicity; allergic reactions; severe eye irritation	Processed foods like beverages, ice cream, candy, baked goods	
Believed safe in food use at low levels	Baked goods, desserts, ice cream, margarine, whipped toppings, frozen fish	
Believed safe in food use at low levels; may cause headaches	Bread, infant formula, processed foods	
Believed safe in food use at low levels	Processed foods like beverages, ice cream, candy, baked goods, chewing gum	Plastics manufacturing

Names	Function	Code	
Acrolein (synthetic; by-product of petroleum)	Starch modifying agent	☹☹	
Adipic acid (from oxidation of cyclohexanol by nitric acid liberating nitrous oxide, a greenhouse gas; on the NIH HSDB)	Neutralizer Buffer	☺?	
Agar (derived from red algae, *Gelidium* Spp.)	Thickener Emulsifier	☺	
Albumin (usually from egg white; may be of ANIMAL origin)	Emulsifier Thickener	☺	
Alcohol (ethanol)	Solvent	☺?	
Algin (also known as alginate)	Stabilizer	☺	
Alginates (extracted from seaweed; ammonium, calcium, potassium, propylene glycol and sodium alginate)	Stabilizer Thickener Emulsifier	☺	
Alginic acid (seaweed extract; on the NIH HSDB)	Vegetable gum Thickener	☺	

Potential Effects	Possible Food Use	Other Uses
Toxic; liver, gastrointestinal, cardiovascular, respiratory, skin and neurotoxicity; suspected carcinogen	Modifier for food starch	Manufacture of agricultural chemicals and plastics
Moderately toxic by ingestion; adverse health effects in animal studies including death; severe eye irritation	Beverages, baked goods, oils, snack foods, processed cheese	Hair color rinse, manufacture of plastics and nylons
Mildly toxic by ingestion; may cause allergic reactions in some people	Ice cream, baked goods, desserts, manufactured meats, jellies	Moisturizer, skin cream, bulk laxative
May cause allergic reactions in some people	Processed foods	Cosmetics
See ethanol	See ethanol	See ethanol
See alginates	See alginates	See alginates
Alginates believed to have beneficial effects on health; alginates inhibited essential nutrient absorption in some animal tests	Beverages, ice cream, desserts, baked goods, candy, cheese spread, salad dressing	Shampoos, hairstyling and perm products, hand lotions and creams
Large amounts may inhibit absorption of essential nutrients	Ice cream, dessert mix, custard mix, flavored milk, cordials, infant formula, yogurt	Toothpaste, skin creams and lotions, antacids

Names	Function	Code
Alitame (synthetic; 2000 times sweeter than sugar; related to aspartame)	Artificial sweetener	☺?
Alkanet (from an herb-like tree root; banned in foods in some countries)	Coloring (red)	☺?
Alkyl sulfates (synthetic alternatives to vegetable fats and oils)	Surfactant	☺?
Allspice (from the dried berries of the allspice tree)	Flavoring	☺
Allura red (FD&C Red No. 40)	Coloring (orange/red)	☹
Allyl heptanoate	Flavoring	☺?
Allyl isothiocyanate (mustard oil from the seeds of the mustard plant; on the Canadian Hotlist)	Flavoring	☺?
Allyl sulfide (found in garlic and horseradish)	Flavoring	☹
Alpha tocopherol (vitamin E; mostly synthetic; may be GE)	Antioxidant Nutrient	☺

Potential Effects	Possible Food Use	Other Uses
Caused reduced body weight gain and increased liver weight in animal studies	Custard mix, jellies, jam, custard powder, ice cream	
Claimed to be harmless, although uncertainties exist	Sausage casing, wines	Cosmetics, hair oil, inks
Not adequately tested for effects on human health; may cause skin irritation	Processed foods	Cosmetics, drugs
Weak sensitizer; may cause skin rash	Processed foods like beverages, ice cream, candy, condiments, baked goods	
See FD&C Red No. 40	See FD&C Red No. 40	See FD&C Red No. 40
Toxic by ingestion; skin irritation	Ice cream, candy, baked goods, candy	
Allergic reactions; skin problems including blistering; regarded as toxic	Processed foods like beverages, ice cream, candy, pickles	Soap, lubricants, manufacture of mustard gas used in warfare
Eye and respiratory tract irritation; liver and kidney damage	Processed foods like beverages, ice cream, candy, baked goods	
May cause the depletion of delta & gamma tocopherol if excess is used in isolation	White flour, white bread, white rice, margarine, dietary supplements	

Names	Function	Code
Aluminum (metal extracted from the mineral ore bauxite; on the NIH HSDB)	Coloring (metallic)	☹
Aluminum ammonium sulfate (ammonium aluminum sulfate; made from ammonium sulfate and aluminum sulfate)	Buffer Neutralizer Firming agent	☺?
Aluminum hydroxide (from bauxite; on the NIH HSDB)	Leavening agent	☺?
Aluminum potassium sulfate (synthetic)	Firming agent Clarifying agent	☺?
Aluminum sulfate (synthetic)	Starch modifying agent	☺?
Amaranth (FD&C Red No 2; the synthetic chemical, not the grain; banned in the USA in 1976)	Coloring (bluish red)	☹☹

Potential Effects	Possible Food Use	Other Uses
Some evidence of links with Alzheimer's disease; lung and kidney disorders; cardiovascular, reproductive and neurotoxicity; the European Parliament said aluminum additives should be banned	External decoration on cakes etc., often added to baking powder, flour, cheese and table salt during manufacture	Face powder, hair coloring, dental fillings, toothpaste, antiperspirant, silver finish to pills and tablets
Ingestion of large doses can cause burning in mouth and throat, vomiting and diarrhea; see aluminum	Baking powder, pickles, relishes, milling and cereal industries	Purification of drinking water, fireproofing, vegetable glue
Ingestion can cause constipation; see aluminum	Baked goods	Antiperspirant, filler in vaccines
Gastrointestinal distress; caused kidney damage and intestinal bleeding in animal studies; see aluminum	Production of various foods including flour, cereal, sugar and cheese	Waterproofing fabrics, sizing paper
Moderately toxic by ingestion; pimples under the arms; allergic reactions; may affect reproduction; see aluminum	Sweet and dill pickles, pickle relish, modifier for food starch	Antiperspirant, deodorant, skin fresheners, packaging materials
See FD&C Red No. 2	See FD&C Red No. 2	See FD&C Red No. 2

Names	Function	Code	
Ambergris (from the intestines of sperm whales; of ANIMAL origin)	Flavoring Fixative	☺	
4-Aminobenzoic acid (PABA; water-soluble "B" group vitamin; on the Canadian Hotlist)	Nutrient additive UV absorber	☺?	
Aminopeptidase (derived from the bacteria *Lactococcus lactis*)	Food enzyme	☺	
Ammonium alginate (ammonium salt of alginic acid extracted from seaweed)	Thickener Stabilizer	☺	
Ammonium aluminum sulfate (aluminum ammonium sulfate)	Buffer Neutralizer Firming agent	☺?	
Ammonium bicarbonate (derived from ammonia and carbon dioxide)	Raising agent Buffer Neutralizer	☺	
Ammonium carbonate (derived from ammonia and carbon dioxide)	Buffer Neutralizer	☺	
Ammonium carrageenan	Stabilizer Thickener	☺?	

Potential Effects	Possible Food Use	Other Uses
Ambergris is 80% cholesterol	Flavoring in foods and beverages	Perfumery
Believed safe in food use at low levels; nausea, diarrhea and liver irritation with excess; photosensitivity; allergic eczema; skin irritation	Dietary supplements	Sunscreen, sunburn creams and lotions
Believed safe in food use, but hasn't been assigned for toxicology literature search	Dairy-based flavoring preparations, cheese manufacture	
See alginates	See alginates	Cosmetics; boiler water
See aluminum ammonium sulfate	See aluminum ammonium sulfate	See aluminum ammonium sulfate
Believed safe in food use at low levels; skin contact can cause rashes on scalp, forehead and hands	Baking powder, cocoa products, chocolate, confections, baked goods	Hair perm solution and cream, fire extinguishers
See ammonium bicarbonate	See ammonium bicarbonate	Hair perm solution and cream
See carrageenan	See carrageenan	

Names	Function	Code
Ammonium chloride (naturally occurring ammonium salt)	Bulking agent	☺?
Ammonium citrate, dibasic & monobasic (ammonium salt of citric acid)	Flavor enhancer Sequestrant	☺
Ammonium furcelleran	Emulsifier Thickener Stabilizer	☺
Ammonium hydroxide (prepared by adding ammonia gas to water; banned in foods in some countries; on the NIH HSDB)	Buffer Neutralizer	☺?
Ammonium persulfate (synthetic)	Preservative Starch modifying agent	☺?
Ammonium phosphate, dibasic and monobasic (salt of phosphoric acid)	Buffer Leavening agent	☺
Ammonium sulfate (synthetic; made from ammonia and sulfuric acid)	Dough conditioner Buffer	☹
Ammonium sulfite (synthetic)	Antioxidant Preservative	☹

Potential Effects	Possible Food Use	Other Uses
Ingestion can cause weight loss, nausea, headache, acidosis and insomnia; contact can cause skin and eye irritation and dermatitis	Flour products, bread, rolls, buns etc, low-sodium dietary foods	Skin wash, eye drops, shampoo, hair perm solution, dyes, metal polish
See citrates	Beverages, fats, oils, ice cream, sauces, soups, jellies	
See furcelleran	See furcelleran	
Toxic by ingestion; respiratory toxicity; poisonous and hazardous when concentrated; severe eye irritation; harmful to the environment	Cocoa products, gelatin	Mascara, hair dye, shampoo, stain remover, cigarettes, food packaging
Skin irritation; respiratory, skin and immunotoxicity; asthma; large oral doses proved fatal to rats	Brewer's yeast, modifier for food starch	Skin lighteners, dyes, cosmetics
Believed safe in food use; has a diuretic effect; makes urine more acidic	Baking powder, beer, ale, stout, bakery foods, purifying sugar	Mouthwash, fireproofing textiles, paper etc.
Gastrointestinal, liver, respiratory and neurotoxicity; fatal to rats in large doses	Bakery products, dough making	Hair perm lotion, tanning industry, fertilizer
See sulfites	Processed foods	Cosmetics, medicines

Names	Function	Code
Amyl acetate (banana oil; synthetic; made from n-amyl alcohol and acetic acid; on the NIH HSDB)	Flavoring Solvent	☹
Amyl alcohol (synthetic; may be made from the hydrocarbon pentane; on the NIH HSDB)	Flavoring Solvent	☹
Amylase (from bacteria or fungi; likely to be GE; may be of ANIMAL origin)	Food enzyme Dough conditioner	☺
Anethole (derived from anise, fennel and others)	Flavoring	☺?
Annatto (dye obtained from the tropical annatto tree)	Coloring (yellow to pink)	☹
Anthocyanins (anthocyanocides; from grape skins or red cabbage)	Coloring (red/violet)	☺☺
Arabinogalactan (larch gum; complex carbohydrate from larch wood; contains high tannic acid levels)	Thickener Stabilizer Emulsifier	☺?

Potential Effects	Possible Food Use	Other Uses
CNS depression; headache; respiratory & neurotoxicity; fatigue; chest pain; mucous membrane irritation	Banana flavoring in processed foods	Perfumes, nail polish, nail polish remover, shoe polish, spray adhesive
Very toxic; narcotic when concentrated; can be absorbed through the skin; small amounts can be fatal	Processed foods like beverages, ice cream, candy, chewing gum	Nail polish, paint, pharmaceutical preparations
Believed safe in food use	Bakery products, bread, flour, modified food starch	Anti-inflammatory in medicine, stain remover
Mouth ulcers; burning sensation in the mouth; skin contact can cause hives and blistering	Processed foods like beverages, ice cream, candy, baked goods	Perfume, toothpaste, mouthwash, denture cream
May cause irritability and head banging in children; hives; hypotension; pruritis; undergoing further testing	Margarine, baked goods, reduced fat spreads, dairy products, breakfast cereals	Fabric dye, soap, varnish, body paints
Considered to have benefits to human health	Soft drinks, jams, ice cream, wines, yogurt, sweets, preserves	Vitamin tablets
Claimed to have beneficial health effects; may cause allergic reactions; tannic acid is thought to be a weak carcinogen	Pudding mixes, beverage bases and mixes, flavor bases, pie filling mixes	Essential oils

Names	Function	Code	
Ascorbic acid (vitamin C; usually made synthetically from d-glucose; may be GE; on the NIH HSDB)	Preservative Antioxidant	☺	
Ascorbyl palmitate (from ascorbic acid and palmitoyl chloride; on the NIH HSDB)	Preservative Antioxidant	☺	
Ascorbyl stearate (fat-soluble ester of vitamin C; may be of ANIMAL origin)	Preservative Antioxidant	☺	
Aspartame (about 200 times sweeter than sugar; prepared from phenylalanine and aspartic acid; breakdown products include methanol, formaldehyde, and formic acid (see all); may be GE)	Artificial sweetener Flavor enhancer	☹	
Azodicarbonamide (from urea and hydrazine; banned in foods in some countries; on the NIH HSDB)	Bleaching agent Maturing agent Oxidizing agent	☺?	
Baker's yeast glycan	Emulsifier Thickener Stabilizer	☺☺	

Potential Effects	Possible Food Use	Other Uses
Vitamin C has beneficial health effects; excessive consumption may cause skin rashes, painful urination and diarrhea	Candy, breakfast cereals, luncheon or deli meats, corned meat	Cosmetic cream, shampoo, hair conditioner, moisturizer
No known adverse effects in humans; retarded growth and bladder stones in rats	Fats and oils, lard, meat and meat by-products, shortening, margarine	Cosmetic creams and lotions, lipstick, pharmaceuticals
No known adverse effects in humans	Processing of foods, fats and oils, lard, shortening, margarine	
Health problems reported to authorities include fatigue, irritability, headache, MS-like symptoms, depression, anxiety, vision problems, dizziness, memory loss, hyperactivity, migraine, aggression & insomnia; not recommended for children or women during pregnancy	Table-top sweeteners, breakfast cereals, beverages, chewing gum, confections; may be added to anything which is "sugar-free" or "without added sugar"	Medications, including those for children
May provoke asthma; has not been adequately tested for effects on human health	Bread, flour, whole wheat flour	Food contact surfaces, plastic manufacturing
Regarded as safe in food use	Cheese spread, sour cream, frozen dessert	

Names	Function	Code
Beeswax, white or yellow (obtained from bees; of ANIMAL origin)	Emulsifier Glazing and polishing agent	☺
Beeswax, bleached	Flavoring	☺
Beeswax, synthetic (a mixture of alcohol esters)	Emulsifier Glazing and polishing agent	☺
Beet red (extracted from beetroot)	Coloring (deep red/purple)	☺
Bentonite (colloidal clay; aluminum silicate; on the NIH HSDB)	Thickener Anti-caking agent	😐?
Benzaldehyde (synthetic almond oil; may be made by the oxidation of toluene; on the NIH HSDB)	Solvent Flavoring	☹☹

Potential Effects	Possible Food Use	Other Uses
May cause mild allergic reactions and contact dermatitis in some people	Candy, unstandardized foods	Mascara, eye makeup, baby cream, lipstick, cosmetics
May cause mild allergic reactions in some people	Processed foods like beverages, ice cream, candy, baked goods	Pharmaceutical ointments, cosmetics, candles
May cause mild allergic reactions and contact dermatitis in some people	Candy, unstandardized foods	Baby lotion, facial cream, diaper rash cream
May contain nitrates so restrict intake in babies and young children	Desserts, jellies, jams, licorice, sweets	Cosmetics
Believed safe in food use; may clog skin pores thus inhibiting proper skin function; see aluminum	Coloring in wine, sugar brewing and purification, settling wine sediments	Cosmetics, facial masks, animal and poultry feeds, detergents
Highly toxic; eye and skin irritation; allergic reactions; convulsions; kidney, liver, respiratory & neurotoxicity; CNS depression; toxic to aquatic organisms	Processed foods like beverages, ice cream, candy, baked goods	Cosmetic cream and lotion, soap, perfume, dye, cigarettes

Names	Function	Code	
Benzene (aromatic hydrocarbon; may be from coal tar, but primarily from petroleum; on the Canadian Hotlist; on the NIH HSDB)	Solvent	☹☹	
Benzoate of soda (sodium benzoate)	Preservative	☹	
Benzoic acid (may be made using phthalic anhydride or toluene; on the NIH HSDB)	Preservative Flavoring	☹	
Benzoin (gum benzoin; from *Styrax* Spp.)	Flavoring Glazing and polishing agent	☺	
Benzophenones (1–12) (a dozen or more different ones exist; on the NIH HSDB)	Flavoring Fixative UV absorber		
Benzoyl peroxide (from benzoyl chloride and sodium or hydrogen peroxide; on the NIH HSDB; on the Canadian Hotlist)	Bleaching agent Maturing agent	☹	
Benzyl acetate (synthetic; obtained from plants, especially jasmine)	Flavoring Solvent	☹	

Potential Effects	Possible Food Use	Other Uses
Cardiovascular, respiratory, gastrointestinal, endocrine, liver, reproductive, immuno, developmental, skin and neurotoxicity; suspected teratogen and mutagen; recognized carcinogen	Food processing, modified hop extract for beer; unsafe levels have been found in some soft drinks that contain vitamin C sodium benzoate and	Paint thinner, nail polish remover, detergents, dyes, pharmaceuticals, adhesives, inks, plastics, resins
See sodium benzoate	See sodium benzoate	See sodium benzoate
Asthma; hives; behavioral problems; hyperactivity; may affect lungs; eye and skin irritation; caution advised if aspirin sensitive; neurotoxicity	Brewed soft drinks, cider, non-dairy dip, chewing gum, fruit juice, tomato ketchup, margarine, ice cream	Cosmetics, hair rinse, skin cleanser, perfume, pharmaceuticals
See gum benzoin	See gum benzoin	
Photoallergic reactions; contact sensitivity; toxic when injected; toxic to aquatic organisms	Synthetic additives for flavorings use in processed foods	Hairspray, hair conditioner, soap, sunscreen, perfume
Allergic reactions; skin irritation; AVOID SKIN CONTACT; high potential for bio-concentration in aquatic organisms	Flour, whole wheat flour, blue cheese, gorgonzola	Manufacture of cosmetics, artificial nail kits, fiberglass resins, pharmaceuticals
Skin and eye irritation; diarrhea; vomiting; liver, gastrointestinal, kidney, and neurotoxicity	Processed foods like beverages, ice cream, candy, baked goods	Perfumes, soap

Names	Function	Code
Benzyl alcohol (synthetically derived from petroleum or coal tar; on the NIH HSDB)	Flavoring Solvent Preservative	☹
Benzyl carbinol (phenethyl alcohol)	Flavoring Preservative	😐?
Benzyl cinnamate (synthetic)	Flavoring	☹
Benzyl salicylate	Flavoring Fixative Solvent	😐?
Bergamot (from bitter orange; *Citrus aurantium*)	Flavoring	😐?
beta-Apo-8'-carotenal (synthetic)	Coloring (orange to yellow/red)	☺☺
beta-Carotene (precursor to vitamin A; made by microbial fermentation of corn and soybean oil; may be GE)	Coloring (yellow or orange)	☺
BHA (butylated hydroxyanisole)	Antioxidant Preservative	☹☹

Potential Effects	Possible Food Use	Other Uses
Headache; skin & mucous membrane irritation; liver and neurotoxicity; contact dermatitis; toxic to aquatic organisms	Processed foods like beverages, ice cream, candy, baked goods	Perfume, shampoo, nail polish remover, fabric softener, cigarettes
Eye irritation; sensitization; toxic if ingested; causes birth defects in rats and CNS injury in mice	Synthetic fruit flavoring in foods	Cosmetics, rose perfumes
Toxic by ingestion; allergic reactions; skin irritation	Processed foods like beverages, ice cream, candy, baked goods	Perfumes
Caution advised if salicylate or aspirin sensitive; photosensitivity	Processed foods like beverages, ice cream, candy, baked goods	Perfumes, sunscreen
Bergamot oil can stain skin brown when exposed to sunlight; photosensitivity	Processed foods like beverages, ice cream, candy, baked goods	Perfumes, hair products for shine
See carotene	Cream cheese spread, smoked fish, cheese slices, bread, butter, processed cheese	
Considered to have many health benefits; partially destroyed by conventional and microwave cooking	Margarine, reduced fat spread, cakes, jams, cheese; dietary supplements	Shampoo, hand and body lotion, lipstick, medicines
See butylated hydroxyanisole	See butylated hydroxyanisole	See butylated hydroxyanisole

Names	Function	Code	
BHT (butylated hydroxytoluene)	Antioxidant Preservative	☹	
Biphenyl (derivative of benzene)	Preservative Anti-fungal	☹	
Boric acid (made by the action of sulfuric or hydrochloric acid on borax; on the Canadian Hotlist; on the NIH HSDB)	Preservative Oral care agent	☹☹	
Borneol (synthetic)	Flavoring	☹	
Bovine rennet (rennin; of ANIMAL origin)	Food enzyme	☺	
Bromates (calcium, potassium, sodium)	Maturing agent Bread improver	☹	
Bromelain (enzyme in pineapple)	Food enzyme	☺	
Brilliant blue FCF (FD&C Blue No. 1)	Coloring (bright blue)	☹	

Potential Effects	Possible Food Use	Other Uses
See butylated hydroxytoluene	See butylated hydroxytoluene	See butylated hydroxytoluene
Nausea; vomiting; irritation of eyes and nose; liver and neurotoxicity; teratogen	Used in packaging citrus fruits, may leave residue, orange marmalade?	
Severe poisonings have occurred after ingestion or application to abraded skin; kidney, cardiovascular, liver reproductive & neurotoxicity	Caviar, fungus control on citrus fruit	Baby powder, bath powder, soap, eye cream, mouthwash, cosmetics
Nausea; vomiting; confusion; dizziness; convulsions	Processed foods like beverages, ice cream, candy, baked goods	Perfumery
See rennet	See rennet	
Respiratory depression; skin eruptions; adverse effects on the CNS and kidney function	Used in making bread	Hair perm neutralizer
Believed to have beneficial health effects; may cause allergic reactions in some	Bread, flour, sausage casings, waffles, meat cuts, pancakes, beer	Skin peels
See FD&C Blue No. 1	See FD&C Blue No. 1	See FD&C Blue No. 1

Names	Function	Code	
Brominated vegetable oil (vegetable oil with bromine added; bromine is toxic; banned in some countries)	Emulsifier Flavor carrier	☹	
Butane (n-butane; from petroleum; on the NIH HSDB)	Propellant Solvent	😐?	
Butanoic acid (butyric acid; synthetic)	Flavoring	☹	
Butyl acetate (synthetic; from acetic acid and butyl alcohol; on the NIH HSDB)	Flavoring Solvent	☹	
Butyl alcohol (synthetic; from benzyl chloride and sodium carbonate)	Flavoring Solvent Clarifying agent	☹	
Butylated hydroxyanisole (BHA; petroleum derivative; from p-methoxyphenol and isobutane; banned in foods in some countries; on the NIH HSDB)	Antioxidant Preservative	☹☹	

Potential Effects	Possible Food Use	Other Uses
Has caused harmful effects in animals including major organ damage, fat deposits in organs and birth defects	Carbonated beverages, ice cream, baked goods, citrus-flavored beverages	
Animal carcinogen; CNS depression; neurotoxicity	Edible vegetable oil-based or lecithin-based pan coatings	Aerosol cosmetics
Gastrointestinal, liver and skin toxicity; caused cancer in animal studies	Processed foods like beverages, ice cream, candy, baked goods	
Gastrointestinal, liver, skin, respiratory & neurotoxicity; conjunctivitis	Processed foods like beverages, ice cream, candy, baked goods	Perfumes, nail polish, nail polish remover, lacquer
Drowsiness, mucous membrane irritation, headache, dizziness; contact dermatitis when applied to the skin	Processed foods like beverages, ice cream, candy, baked goods	Shampoo, perfumery, waxes, resins, shellac
Hives; hay fever; headache; wheezing; fatigue; asthma; may affect kidneys, thyroid, stomach, and reproduction; hormone disruption; NRC; endocrine, gastrointestinal, liver, respiratory, skin, immuno and neurotoxicity, animal carcinogen;	Fats and oils, lard, shortening, instant mashed potatoes, reduced fat spread, margarine, processed meats, ice cream	Cosmetics, hair dressings, eye shadow, lipstick, mascara, pet foods, food packaging

Names	Function	Code	
Butylated hydroxytoluene (BHT; petroleum derivative; banned in foods in some countries; on the NIH HSDB)	Antioxidant Preservative	☹	
Butylene glycol (1,3-butanediol; synthetic; on the NIH HSDB)	Humectant Solvent	☹	
Butyraldehyde (synthetic)	Flavoring	☺?	
Caffeine (obtained as a by-product of decaffination; psychoactive drug)	Flavoring Stimulant	☹	
Caffeine Citrate	Flavoring	☹	
Calcium acetate (elemental calcium bound to acetic acid)	Food acid Firming agent	☺☺	

Potential Effects	Possible Food Use	Other Uses
Chronic hives; dermatitis; fatigue; asthma; aggressive behavior; bronchospasm; may affect stomach, liver, kidneys and reproduction; NRC; possible carcinogen; toxic to aquatic organisms	Edible fats and oils, chewing gum, fish products, dry breakfast cereals, beer and malt drinks, polyethylene film for wrapping food	Shaving cream, baby oil, baby lotion, lipstick, eyeliner, pet foods, packaging materials, rubber, jet fuel
Severe eye irritation; ingestion can cause kidney damage, drowsiness, vomiting, depression, coma and death; may be harmful to the environment	Processed foods	Hairspray, setting lotion, shampoo, mascara, deicing aircraft
Respiratory & skin toxicity; possible irritant & narcotic	Processed foods like beverages, ice cream, candy, baked goods	Making rubber, plasticizers and resins
Cardiovascular, respiratory, kidney, gastrointestinal, musculoskeletal, liver, and neurotoxicity; insomnia; nervousness; hyperactivity; irritability; migraine; birth defects; infertility; NRC	Cola-type beverages, root beer beverages, some processed foods	Lipstick
See caffeine and citrates	See caffeine	
Believed safe in food use; low oral toxicity	Beer, ale, bread, pickles, cheese	Dyeing and curing skins, cosmetic fragrance

Names	Function	Code	
Calcium alginate (calcium salt of alginic acid extracted from seaweed)	Thickener Stabilizer	☺	
Calcium aluminum silicate (contains aluminum)	Anti-caking agent	☺?	
Calcium ascorbate (prepared from ascorbic acid and calcium carbonate)	Preservative Antioxidant	☺☺	
Calcium benzoate (calcium salt of benzoic acid)	Preservative	☹	
Calcium carbonate (crushed chalk, limestone, marble, dolomite, coral; on the NIH HSDB)	Coloring (white) Firming agent	☺	
Calcium carrageenan	Thickener Emulsifier	☺?	
Calcium chloride (chloride salt of calcium)	Firming agent Sequestrant	☺	
Calcium citrate (prepared from citrus fruits)	Buffer Sequestrant Yeast food	☺	

Potential Effects	Possible Food Use	Other Uses
See alginates	See alginates	Hand lotion and cream, shampoo, hair perms
Believed safe in food use at low levels?; see aluminum	Garlic salt, onion salt, table salt, vanilla powder	
Believed safe in food use at low levels	Concentrated milk products, cooked and cured meat products, canned mushrooms, canned tuna, beer	
Asthma; hives; anaphylaxis; hyperactivity; behavioral problems; eczema; caution advised if aspirin sensitive; NRC	Brewed soft drinks, non-dairy dip, chewing gum, fruit juice, margarine, ice cream	
Believed safe in food use at low levels; excess can cause abdominal pain, nausea and constipation	Bread, cookies, crackers, cakes, candy, ice cream, sweets, canned fruit and vegetables	Cosmetics, face powder, cigarettes, toothpaste
See carrageenan	See carrageenan	Toothpaste
Believed safe in food use at low levels; stomach upsets; irritation of skin and mucous membranes; irregular heartbeat	Cottage cheese, jellies, canned tomatoes, low sodium salt substitute	Cosmetics, eye lotion, fire extinguishers
See citrates	Candy, jellies, jams, bakery products, processed cheese, canned vegetables	

Names	Function	Code	
Calcium disodium EDTA (calcium disodium ethylenediamine tetraacetic acid (or tetraacetate); banned in foods in some countries)	Preservative Sequestrant	☹	
Calcium fumarate (calcium bound to fumaric acid)	Acidifier Antioxidant	☺☺	
Calcium furcelleran	Emulsifier Thickener Stabilizer	☺?	
Calcium glycerophosphate (calcium GP; contains calcium and phosphorus)	Stabilizer Nutrient additive	☺☺	
Calcium hydroxide (slaked lime; by the hydration of lime; on the NIH HSDB)	Neutralizer Firming agent	☺	
Calcium iodate (contains iodine; iodine is on the Canadian Hotlist)	Dough conditioner Germicide	☺?	
Calcium lactate (may be of ANIMAL origin)	Buffer Firming agent Yeast food	☺?	

Potential Effects	Possible Food Use	Other Uses
Muscle cramps; blood in the urine; intestinal upset; kidney damage; mineral imbalance; chromosome damage; may increase the uptake of heavy metals; may affect liver and reproduction	Dressings, soft drinks, sandwich spreads, beer, ale, margarine, instant teas	Used medically to detoxify heavy metal poisoning
See fumaric acid	See fumaric acid	
See furcelleran	See furcelleran	
Believed safe in food use	Unstandardized dessert mixes, baking powder, dietary supplements	Toothpaste
Believed safe in food use; toxic and hazardous in concentrated form	Canned peas, fruit products, infant formula, beer, ale	Depilatories, skin cream, pesticides
Believed safe in food use at low levels; may cause allergic reactions; advise caution if thyroid imbalance	Bread, bakery products, table salt	Deodorant
Believed safe in food use; may cause stomach upset and cardiac disturbance; people with intolerance to lactose may wish to avoid	Candy, baking powder, canned bean sprouts, canned peas, canned grapefruit, condensed milk	Dentifrices, animal feeds; if found in oral menstrual relief products, unsafe

Names	Function	Code
Calcium oxide (quick lime; strongly caustic; made from limestone; on the NIH HSDB)	Dough conditioner Yeast food pH adjusting agent	☺?
Calcium peroxide (from calcium hydroxide & sodium peroxide; on the NIH HSDB)	Bleaching agent Dough conditioner Starch modifying agent	☺?
Calcium phosphate, tribasic (from phosphoric acid and calcium oxide or calcium nitrate; on the NIH HSDB)	Buffer Sequestrant	☺
Calcium phytate (calcium salt of phytic acid; may be from corn; may be GE	Sequestrant	☺
Calcium propionate (calcium salt of propionic acid)	Preservative Mold inhibitor	☺?
Calcium silicate (made from lime and diatomaceous earth; on the NIH HSDB)	Anti-caking agent Glazing agent	☺

Potential Effects	Possible Food Use	Other Uses
Believed safe in food use; can cause severe damage to skin and mucous membranes on contact; thermal and chemical burns	Flour products, bread, buns, soup, malted milk powder, canned peas, sour cream, processing tripe, confections	Cosmetics, home and garden pesticides, insecticides, plaster
Believed safe in food use; can cause skin irritation; requires further testing for safe use as a food additive	Bread, bakery products, edible oils, modified starch	Toothpaste, disinfectant for seeds, waste water treatment
Believed safe in food use; can cause skin and eye irritation on contact	Flour products, malted milk powder, cereal flours, condiments	Toothpaste, baby powder, tooth powder, fertilizer
Believed safe in food use; claimed to have beneficial effects on health	Glazed fruit	
Learning difficulties; fatigue; irritability; headache; gastric irritation; aggression; asthma; sensitivity to propionates occurs in conjunction with sensitivity to other preservatives	Bread, processed cheese, poultry stuffing, chocolate products	Cosmetics, anti-fungal medication
Believed safe in food use; inhalation may cause respiratory tract irritation; asthma	Baking powder, rice, chewing gum, table salt, vanilla powder	Face powder, eye shadow, lime glass, antibiotics

Names	Function	Code	
Calcium sorbate (synthetic; derived from sorbic acid)	Preservative	☺?	
Calcium stearate (synthetic; calcium bound to stearic acid; may be of ANIMAL origin; may be GE)	Anti-caking agent Release agent Emulsifier	☺☺	
Calcium stearoyl-2-lactylate (calcium salt of lactyl lactate; may be of ANIMAL origin)	Dough conditioner Whipping agent	☺	
Calcium sulfate (Plaster of Paris; made from gypsum; on the NIH HSDB)	Dough conditioner Firming agent	☺	
Calcium tartrate (derived from cream of tartar or from wine dregs)	Emulsifier Thickener Stabilizer	☺☺	
Camphor (may be from laurel trees; usually synthetic from pinene isolated from turpentine; on the Canadian Hotlist; on the NIH HSDB)	Flavoring Preservative Plasticizer	☹	
Candelilla wax (from the candelilla plant, *Euphorbia cerifera*)	Glazing agent Emollient	☺☺	
Canola oil (rapeseed oil; likely to be GE)	Emulsifier	☹	

Potential Effects	Possible Food Use	Other Uses
Contact hives; asthma; skin irritation; allergic reactions; behavioral problems	Bread, cheese products, soft drinks, chocolate syrup, cheesecake	Ointments, cosmetics
Believed safe in food use	Salt, garlic salt, dietary supplements, candy	Hair-grooming products, making Crayons & pencils
Believed safe in food use; adverse reactions have occurred in animals during testing	Bread, cake mix, dried egg white, instant mashed potatoes	Cosmetic powders
Believed safe in food use; large amounts may cause intestinal obstruction and constipation	Flour, baking powder, cereal flours, canned tomatoes, blue cheese, making tofu (Japan)	Toothpastes and powders, brewing industry, plaster casts
Believed safe in food use	Cookies, crackers, unstandardized foods	Tobacco
Toxic by ingestion and skin absorption; gastrointestinal respiratory, skin, liver, and neurotoxicity; especially avoid during pregnancy	Beverages, baked goods, condiments	Deodorant, depilatories, eye lotions, skin cream, lacquers and varnishes
Believed safe in food use	Coating for foods, chewing gum	Lipstick, writing inks, mascara, cosmetics
See rapeseed oil	Salad oils, cooking oils, cake mixes	Insect spray

Names	Function	Code
Canthaxanthin (usually from beta carotene but may be of ANIMAL origin; banned in some countries)	Coloring (pink)	☺?
Caprenin (synthetic; contains behenic acid from hydrogenated rapeseed oil)	Fat substitute	☺?
Caramel (burnt sugar; may be from sugar beet, sugar cane or corn syrup; may be GE; on the NIH HSDB)	Coloring (dark brown) Flavoring	😐?
Caramel color III (may be from sugar beet, sugar cane or maize starch; made using ammonia; may be GE)	Coloring (dark brown to black) Flavoring	☹
Carbon black (synthetic; may be of ANIMAL origin; banned in foods in some countries; on the NIH HSDB)	Coloring (black)	☺?
Carbon dioxide (commercially produced by fermentation; on the NIH HSDB)	Propellant Carbonation Preservative	☺
Carboxymethyl cellulose (made from cotton by-products; may be GE)	Thickener Stabilizer Emulsifier	☹

Potential Effects	Possible Food Use	Other Uses
Loss of night vision; skin discoloration; sensitivity to glare; recurrent hives; "gold dust" retinopathy	Fish sticks, ice cream, crackers, pickles, sauces, preserves	Artificial skin tanning pills, oral drugs
Behenic acid is poorly digested and may increase cholesterol levels; see rapeseed oil	Substitute for cocoa butter used in candy bars	
Gastrointestinal problems; requires tests for sub-acute, mutagenic, teratogenic and reproductive effects	Brown bread, cola drinks, chocolate, ice cream, jams, candy, syrups, baked goods	Cosmetics, skin lotions, pet foods mouthwash, toothpaste
May affect reproduction, liver, and stomach; hyperactivity; caused blood toxicity and convulsions in animal tests	Jams, soy sauce, oyster sauce, cookies, crackers, pickles, dark bread, chocolate coating, dark beers	Pet foods
Skin and respiratory irritation; recognized carcinogen	Candy	Eye cosmetics, shoe polish, printing ink
Believed safe in food use; may reduce fertility; neurotoxicity; suspected teratogen	Carbonated beverages, gassed cream	"Smoke" or "fog" stage effects, dry ice
Poorly absorbed; flatulence; large amounts can cause diarrhea and abdominal cramps; caused cancer and tumors in animal studies	Infant formula, ice cream, icings, candy, cottage cheese, cream cheese spread	Hair setting lotion, laxatives, hand cream, antacids, tobacco

Names	Function	Code
Carmine (aluminum lake of carminic acid; on the NIH HSDB)	Coloring (red)	☹
Carminic acid (active coloring from cochineal; restricted in some countries)	Coloring (red)	☹
Carnauba wax (from the Brazilian wax palm, *Copernicia cerifera*)	Glazing agent Texturiser	☺
Carob bean gum (locust bean gum)	Thickener Stabilizer Emulsifier	☺
Carotene (precursor to vitamin A; mostly of plant origin; may be of ANIMAL origin; may be GE)	Coloring (yellow or orange)	☺
Carrageenan (extract of red seaweed; may be degraded, un-degraded or native; may contain or create MSG)	Thickener Stabilizer Emulsifier	😐?
Carvacrol (synthetic)	Flavoring	😐?
Casein (phosphoprotein found in cows milk)	Thickener Texturiser	😐?

Potential Effects	Possible Food Use	Other Uses
See cochineal	See cochineal	Cosmetic colors
See cochineal	See cochineal	Mascara, blush, eye shadow
Rarely causes allergic reactions; contact dermatitis; gastric irritation	Candy, waxed fruit (to maintain freshness and appeal), fruit juice, sauces	Cosmetics, lipstick, mascara, car polish
See locust bean gum	See locust bean gum	See locust bean gum
Considered to have many health benefits; partially destroyed by conventional and microwave cooking	Margarine, dairy blend, reduced fat spread, cakes, jams, cheese, dietary supplements	Skin care products, cosmetics, cigarettes
May affect gastrointestinal tract; stomach; NRC; ulcerative colitis; suspected carcinogen when degraded	Ice cream, cake mix, candy, pastries, cookies, crackers, chocolate products, infant formula	Pet foods, cosmetics, cough medicines, toothpaste
Ingestion can cause cardiac failure, respiratory and circulatory depression	Processed foods like beverages, ice cream, candy, baked goods	Disinfectant, mouthwash
Allergic reactions; may exacerbate symptoms of autism; may increase levels of cholesterol	Ice cream, fruit sherbet, special diet preparations	Beauty masks, depilatories, hair care products

Names	Function	Code	
Castor oil (oil from seeds of the castor bean, Ricinus communis; on the NIH HSDB)	Flavoring Release agent	😐?	
Catalase (from fungi or bovine liver; may be of ANIMAL origin; probably GE; on the Canadian Hotlist)	Food enzyme Antioxidant	☺	
Cellulase (from the fungi *Aspergillus niger* or Trichoderma reesei; probably GE)	Food enzyme	☺	
Cellulose (fiber from plants; insoluble dietary fiber; may be GE)	Anti-caking agent Emulsifier	☺☺	
Cellulose gums	Thickener Stabilizer Emulsifier	☹	
Cellulose, microcrystalline (colloidal crystalline part of cellulose; may be GE)	Thickener Stabilizer Filler	😐?	
Chlorine (poisonous irritating gas; made by electrolysis; on the Canadian Hotlist; on the NIH HSDB)	Bleaching and oxidizing agent Preservative	☹	
Chlorine dioxide (poisonous pungent gas)	Flour treatment agent	☹	

Potential Effects	Possible Food Use	Other Uses
Pelvic congestion; ingestion can induce abortion; eye & skin irritation; intestinal tract irritation; possible allergen	Candy, candy, beverages, ice cream	Eye pencil, body wash, cosmetics, pharmaceutical laxatives
Believed safe in food use	Cheese manufacture, spice extracts, soft drinks, treatment of food wrappers	Oral antioxidant formulas
Believed safe in food use	Spice extract, liquid coffee concentrate, shrimp and clam processing	Laundry detergent
Believed safe in food use	Grated or shredded cheese	Cosmetic creams, mascara
See carboxymethylcellulose	See carboxymethylcellulose	Hand creams and lotions
Not recommended for infants and young children; no longer listed as GRAS	Frozen desserts, sherbet, grated or shredded cheese	Nail enamel, emulsions, wood filler
Respiratory, kidney, skin, gastrointestinal, liver and neurotoxicity; hazardous to water organisms	Flour, whole wheat flour	Bleaches, paints, plastics, solvents, disinfectants
Respiratory, reproductive, developmental and skin toxicity; destroys vitamin E; toxic to water organisms	Flour, whole wheat flour	Pulp and paper manufacture, poultry processing

Names	Function	Code
Chloropentafluoroethane	Aerating agent	☺?
Chlorophyll (green pigment in plants)	Coloring (olive to dark green)	☺
Cholecalciferol (vitamin D3; synthetically made using irradiation; may be GE; on the NIH HSDB)	Nutrient additive	☺
Choline bitartrate (choline ('B' group vitamin) bound to tartaric acid)	Nutrient additive	☺
Chymosin (A & B) (rennin; from calf stomach or fungi or bacteria; may be of ANIMAL origin; probably GE)	Food enzyme	☺
Cinnamaldehyde (synthetic; from a wood-rotting fungus or from benzaldehyde and acetaldehyde; on the NIH HSDB)	Flavoring	☹
Cinnamic acid (cinoxate)	Flavoring UV absorber	☺?
Cinnamyl alcohol (synthetic)	Flavoring	☺

Potential Effects	Possible Food Use	Other Uses
Cardiovascular and neurotoxicity	Unstandardized foods	Electrical insulation
Believed to have beneficial effects on health; can cause a sensitivity to light	Soups, sauces, olive oil, soybean oil, ice cream, pickles, ketchup	Antiperspirant, deodorant, mouthwash
Believed to have beneficial effects on health; excess can cause serious health problems	Breakfast cereals, milk products, margarine	Baby oil, bath and shower gel
Choline has many beneficial effects on health; excess can cause diarrhea	Dietary supplements	
Believed safe in food use	Cheddar cheese, cream cheese, cottage cheese, sour cream	
Allergic reactions; hives; skin de-pigmentation; skin and mucous membrane irritation; lip swelling	Processed foods like beverages, ice cream, candy, baked goods, condiments	Perfume, soap mouthwash, toothpaste, medicines
Allergic skin rashes; photoallergic reactions	Processed foods like beverages, ice cream, candy, baked goods	Sunscreen, perfume
May cause allergic reactions in some people	Processed foods like beverages, ice cream, candy, baked goods	Perfume, deodorant

Names	Function	Code	
Citrates (salts of citric acid; potassium, ammonium, calcium, sodium, manganese, isopropyl, lecithin, caffeine, magnesium, stearyl, triethyl)	Flavor enhancer Sequestrant Emulsifier Buffer	☺	
Citric acid (may be extracted from citrus fruits or made synthetically by mold fermentation of carbohydrates; may be GE; on the NIH HSDB)	Acidulant Flavoring Preservative	☺	
Citronella oil (extract from fresh grass; 93% geraniol)	Flavoring Fragrance	☺?	
Citrus red No. 2 (monoazo dye; banned in some countries)	Coloring (red)	☹	
Cochineal (dried bodies of female insect *Coccus cacti*; of ANIMAL origin; restricted in some countries)	Coloring (red)	☹	
Copper gluconate (copper bound to gluconic acid)	Characterization	☺☺	

Potential Effects	Possible Food Use	Other Uses
Believed safe in food use; citrates may interfere with the results of medical laboratory tests for liver function, pancreatic function and blood pH level	Various processed foods	
Believed safe in food use; may provoke symptoms in those who react to MSG; may aggravate the herpes simplex virus; excess may lead to tooth erosion	Cookies, crackers, cheese, ice cream, jams, jellies, processed cheese, soft drinks, fruit drinks, infant formula	Freckle cream, eye drops, nail bleaches, skin fresheners, hair rinses, shampoo
Gastrointestinal irritation; allergic reactions; asthma; skin rash; hay fever	Processed foods like beverages, ice cream, candy, baked goods	Soap, cosmetics, perfume, insect repellant
Allergic reactions; caused adverse health effects in animal studies including organ damage and cancer	Authorized for use only on the skins of whole oranges, possibly found in orange marmalade	
Anaphylaxis (possibly life-threatening); asthma; hives; hay fever; caution advised if aspirin sensitive	Some alcoholic drinks, red applesauce, pie fillings, meats, baked goods, yogurt	Eye makeup, medicines, pet food, shampoo, photography
Believed safe in food use	Dietary supplements	Animal feeds, breath freshener products

Names	Function	Code
Corn oil (may be GE)	Emulsifier Texturiser Emollient	😐?
Corn starch (may be GE)	Thickener Release agent	😐?
Corn syrup (syrup prepared from corn starch; may be GE)	Sweetener Flavoring	😊
Cream of Tartar (may be from argols or synthetic from tartaric acid)	Buffer Stabilizer	😐?
Cyclamates (calcium, potassium and sodium; break down to cyclohexlyamine and other chemical compounds; banned from foods in the USA in 1969)	Artificial sweetener	😟😦
Cysteine hydrochloride (L-cysteine (essential amino acid) bound to hydrochloric acid; may be GE)	Nutrient additive Raising agent	😊
Decanal (synthetic)	Flavoring	😐?
Desoxycholic acid	Emulsifier	😐?

Potential Effects	Possible Food Use	Other Uses
Allergic reactions in some people; skin irritation; caused birth defects in animal studies	Salad oil, mayonnaise, bakery products	Cosmetic cream, body wash, toothpaste
Allergic reactions; asthma; skin rash; hay fever	Used on food containers to prevent sticking	Dusting powder
Believed safe in food use; can cause allergic reactions in some people	Processed foods like beverages, ice cream, candy, baked goods	Cosmetics, aspirin, stamps
People with impaired kidney or liver function, high blood pressure, edema or heart problems may wish to avoid	Baking powder, honey wine	
Cyclohexylamine may cause cardiovascular, respiratory, reproductive, immuno and neurotoxicity; caused numerous adverse effects in animal studies	Currently banned in foods in the USA and Canada, although attempts are now being made to allow them to be reintroduced	
Has a number of health benefits; may exacerbate thrush; those with diabetes mellitus use with caution	Dietary supplements, unstandardized bakery foods, bread, flour	Shampoo, skin cream
Eye and skin irritation; toxic by ingestion	Processed foods like beverages, ice cream, candy, baked goods	
Toxic by ingestion; caused tumors in animal studies	Dried egg whites	

Names	Function	Code	
Dextrans (complex carbohydrates produced by bacteria; may be GE)	Foam stabilizer Thickener	☺?	
Dextrin (produced from starch from wheat or corn; probably GE)	Thickener Foam stabilizer	☺	
Dextrose (from corn; probably GE)	Sweetener	☺	
Dichloromethane (methylene chloride)	Carrier or extraction solvent	☹☹	
Dichlorvos (organophosphate insecticide; on the NIH HSDB)	Pesticide	☹☹	
Dimethylpolysiloxane (synthetic; contains silicone)	Antifoaming agent	☺?	
Dioctyl sodium sulfosuccinate (synthetic; from alcohol, malic anhydride and sodium bisulfite; on the NIH HSDB)	Wetting agent Processing aid	☺?	
Dipotassium phosphate (potassium bound to phosphorus)	Buffer Sequestrant	☺	

Potential Effects	Possible Food Use	Other Uses
Believed safe in food use; caused cancer in animals when injected	Beer, soft-centered candies, as an alternative to barley malt	Cuticle removers
Believed safe in foods; allergic reactions in some people; people with celiac disease should avoid	Cereals, beer	Matches
See corn syrup	See corn syrup	See corn syrup
See methylene chloride	See methylene chloride	See methylene chloride
Reproductive, immuno, skin, gastrointestinal, liver, developmental, blood and neurotoxicity; recognized carcinogen and teratogen	Sprayed on tomatoes, radishes, lettuce and mushrooms, used on food packaging	Agricultural use, pet flea and tick collars, insect sprays, pest strips
Acute or delayed hypersensitivity reactions; nausea; diarrhea	Jam, fats and oils for frying, soft drinks, soups, milk	Ointment base, topical drugs, protective cream
Skin & mucous membrane irritation; tissue damage; undergoing further evaluation for safety	Sausage casings, gums, cocoa, sauces, beverages, sugar industry	Hair styling products, detergents, laxatives
Believed safe in food use; may reduce mineral absorption	Nondairy powdered coffee creamer, cheese	Nail varnish, detergent

Names	Function	Code	
Disodium EDTA (disodium ethylenediamine tetraacetic acid (or tetraacetate))	Preservative Sequestrant	☹	
Disodium guanylate (often used in combination with MSG)	Flavor enhancer	☺?	
Disodium inosinate (of ANIMAL origin; often contains MSG)	Flavor enhancer	☺?	
Disodium phosphate (may be made from dicalcium phosphate (or phosphoric acid) and soda ash; on the NIH HSDB)	Buffer Emulsifier Sequestrant	☺	
Dodecyl gallate (ester of gallic acid derived from tannin)	Antioxidant	☹	
EDTA (ethylene diamine tetraacetic acid)	Sequestrant Preservative	☺?	
EDTA calcium disodium	Sequestrant	☹	

Potential Effects	Possible Food Use	Other Uses
See ethylenediamine tetraacetic acid	Canned potatoes, dried banana products, sauces, sandwich spreads, dressings	Deodorant, body wash, shampoo, skin cream
Caution advised if aspirin sensitive; people with gout or uric acid kidney stones may wish to avoid; NRC	Canned foods, sauces, snack foods, soups	
People with gout or uric acid kidney stones may wish to avoid; kidney problems; NRC	Canned vegetables	
Believed safe in food use; those with impaired kidney function may wish to avoid; mild skin irritation	Cheese, evaporated milk, beverages, sauces, chocolate products	Shampoo, hair color, deodorant soap, detergents
Allergic reactions; contact dermatitis; gastric irritation; caution advised if aspirin sensitive; NRC; caused pathological changes in the spleen, kidneys and liver in animal studies	Dairy blend, edible fats and oils, reduced fat spread, margarine	Cosmetic cream, ink
See ethylene diamine tetraacetic acid	See ethylene diamine tetraacetic acid	See ethylene diamine tetraacetic acid
See calcium disodium EDTA	See calcium disodium EDTA	See calcium disodium EDTA

Names	Function	Code	
EDTA disodium	Sequestrant	☹	
Epichlorohydrin	Starch modifying agent Solvent	☹☹	
Erythorbic acid (iso-ascorbic acid; produced from sugar; may be from corn; may be GE; on the NIH HSDB)	Antioxidant Preservative	☺	
Erythritol (type of sugar alcohol derived from algae and lichens)	Sweetener Humectant	☺☺	
Erythromycin (derived from the bacteria *Streptomyces erythreus*)	Antibacterial	☹	
Erythrosine (FD&C Red No. 3)	Coloring	☹	
Estradiol (estrogen hormone; on the Canadian Hotlist)	Animal hormonal implant	☹	

Potential Effects	Possible Food Use	Other Uses
See disodium EDTA	See disodium EDTA	
Cardiovascular, endocrine, reproductive, kidney, liver, developmental, respiratory, gastrointestinal, immuno & neurotoxicity; sensitizer; recognized carcinogen	Modifier for food starch	Paper coating, coatings on the insides of cans, printing, wood stain and varnish
May cause allergic reactions in some people; has only 5% of the vitamin capacity of ascorbic acid	Breakfast cereal, beverages, flour products, candy, lunchmeat products	Cosmetics
Believed safe in food use at low levels	Processed foods, substitute for sugar	Moisturizing creams and lotions
Allergic reactions; may lead to antibiotic resistance in humans	May be residual in beef, pork, turkey meat, milk, eggs	Animal feeds
See FD&C Red No. 3	See FD&C Red No. 3	
Elevated levels of estradiol can lead to many adverse health effects in both sexes	May be residual in meat products, especially beef and lamb	Perfumes, hormone creams and lotions

Names	Function	Code
Ethanol (ethyl alcohol)	Solvent	☺?
Ethoxyquin (synthetic antioxidant; 6-ethoxy-1, 2-dihydro-2, 2,4-trimethylquinoline; banned in foods in some countries)	Antioxidant	☹
Ethyl acetate (synthetic; on the NIH HSDB)	Flavoring Solvent	☹
Ethyl acrylate (synthetic; may be from acetaldehyde, ethanol and acetic acid; on the NIH HSDB)	Flavoring	☹☹
Ethyl alcohol (ethanol)	Solvent	☺?
Ethyl beta-apo-8'-carotenoate	Coloring	☺☺

Potential Effects	Possible Food Use	Other Uses
Toxic in large amounts or if denatured; implicated in mouth, throat and tongue cancers; cardiovascular, developmental, endocrine, liver, gastrointestinal and reproductive toxicity	Processed foods like ice cream, candy, baked goods, alcoholic beverages	Mouthwash, nail polish, anti-acne cream, perfumes, bubble bath, aftershave lotion, antifreeze
Skin and immunotoxicity; has caused adverse health effects in animals including skin, thyroid, reproductive and kidney problems	Paprika, ground chili powder	Pet foods
Respiratory, skin and neurotoxicity; CNS depression; skin irritation	Processed foods like beverages, ice cream, candy, baked goods	Perfumes, nail polish, nail polish remover
Gastrointestinal, liver, skin, kidney, developmental, respiratory & neurotoxicity; animal carcinogen	Processed foods like beverages, ice cream, candy, baked goods	Adhesives in carpet resins, printing industry, semiconductors
See ethanol	See ethanol	
See beta-apo-8'-carotenal	See beta-apo-8'-carotenal	

Names	Function	Code
Ethylenediamine tetraacetic acid (EDTA; synthetic amino acid; on the NIH HSDB)	Sequestrant Preservative	☹
Ethylene oxide (gas derived from ethylene; banned in food use in some countries; on the Canadian Hotlist; on the NIH HSDB)	Fumigant	☹☹
Ethyl formate (synthetic)	Flavoring Anti-mycotic agent	😐?
Ethyl maltol (synthetic; may be from corn or wheat; probably GE)	Flavoring Processing aid	☺
Ethyl methyl phenylglycidate (synthetic)	Flavoring	😐?
Ethyl myristate (ethyl alcohol and myristic acid; may be of ANIMAL origin)	Flavoring Emollient	☺

Potential Effects	Possible Food Use	Other Uses
Asthma; allergic reactions; skin rash; kidney damage; believed to have health benefits when used in chelation therapy; on a list of additives to be studied for toxicity; toxic to aquatic organisms	Soft drinks	Shampoo, bar soaps, shower gel, cosmetics, dishwashing liquid, hair color, pharmaceuticals
Asthma; reproductive, liver, respiratory, developmental, gastrointestinal, immuno, kidney, skin & neurotoxicity; recognized carcinogen; toxic to aquatic organisms	Whole and ground spices; processed seasonings	Disinfectants, insecticides
Neurotoxicity; skin and mucous membrane irritation; narcotic in high concentrations	Processed foods like beverages, ice cream, candy, baked goods, dried fruits	Tobacco
Believed safe in food use; moderately toxic when injected	Wines, chocolate, desserts	
Caused adverse health effects in animal studies including testicular atrophy	Processed foods like beverages, ice cream, candy, baked goods	
Believed safe in cosmetic use; some myristates can promote acne	Processed foods like beverages, ice cream, candy, baked goods	Cosmetics, cigarettes

Names	Function	Code	
Ethyl palmitate (may be of ANIMAL origin)	Flavoring Emollient	☺	
Ethyl salicylate (synthetic)	Flavoring	☺?	
Ethyl vanillin (synthetic; see also vanillin)	Flavoring	☺?	
Eucalyptus oil (dinkum oil; from the fresh leaves of the eucalyptus tree)	Flavoring Local antiseptic	☺?	
Farnesol (synthetic)	Flavoring	☺?	
Fast Green FCF (FD&C Green No. 3)	Coloring (sea green)	☹	
FD&C Blue No. 1 (brilliant blue; synthetic; coal tar dye; banned in foods in some countries)	Coloring (bright blue)	☹	
FD&C Blue No. 1 Aluminum Lake (may contain aluminum)	Coloring	☹	
FD&C Blue No. 2 (indigotin; synthetic; coal tar dye; banned in foods in some countries)	Coloring (moderate bright green)	☹	

Potential Effects	Possible Food Use	Other Uses
Believed safe in cosmetic use; some palmitates can cause contact dermatitis	Processed foods like beverages, ice cream, candy, baked goods	Cosmetics, cigarettes
Allergic reactions; caution advised if aspirin sensitive; may adversely interact with some medications	Processed foods like beverages, ice cream, candy, baked goods	Perfumes
Caused adverse health effects in animal studies; skin irritation	Processed foods like beverages, ice cream, candy, baked goods	Perfumes
Can cause allergic reactions and skin irritation; large oral doses (1 tsp) can be fatal	Processed foods like beverages, ice cream, candy, baked goods	Skin fresheners, shampoo, skin cream, makeup
Mildly toxic by ingestion; animal mutagen	Processed foods like beverages, ice cream, candy, baked goods	Perfumes
See FD&C Green No. 3	See FD&C Green No. 3	See FD&C Green No. 3
Asthma; hives; hay fever; allergic reactions; NRC; caution advised if aspirin sensitive; caused tumors in animal studies	Gelatin, feta cheese, canned processed peas, desserts, soft drinks, dairy products, cereals	Toothpaste, pet foods, cosmetics, hair dye, deodorant
See FD&C Blue No. 1; see also aluminum	Candy, candy, decorating eggshells	Cosmetics; pet foods, drugs
Asthma; allergic reactions; hyperactivity; NRC; heart problems; carcinogenic	Bottled soft drinks, ice cream, candy, bakery products, candy	Pet foods

Names	Function	Code	
FD&C Blue No. 2 Aluminum Lake (may contain aluminum)	Coloring	☹	
FD&C Green No. 3 (fast green FCF; synthetic; banned in foods in some countries)	Coloring (sea green)	☹	
FD&C Green No. 3 Aluminum Lake (may contain aluminum)	Coloring	☹	
FD&C Green No. 3 Calcium Lake (synthetic)	Coloring	☹	
FD&C Red No. 2 (amaranth; synthetic; coal tar and azo dye; banned in foods in some countries including the USA)	Coloring (bluish red)	☹☹	
FD&C Red No. 3 (erythrosine; synthetic; coal tar dye; banned in foods in some countries)	Coloring (bluish pink)	☹	
FD&C Red No. 40 (allura red ac; synthetic; coal tar dye; from naphthalene and toluene compounds; banned in foods in some countries)	Coloring (orange/red)	☹	

Potential Effects	Possible Food Use	Other Uses
See FD&C Blue No. 2; see also aluminum	Candy, candy, decorating eggshells	Pet foods
Sensitization in allergenic people; cause bladder and malignant tumors in animal studies	Processed foods like beverages, ice cream, candy, baked goods, jam, ketchup	Pet foods, body wash, cosmetics (except near the eyes)
See FD&C Green No. 3; see also aluminum	Candy, candy, decorating eggshells	Pet foods
See FD&C Green No. 3	Candy, candy, decorating eggshells	Pet foods
May affect reproduction, kidneys and liver; asthma; hives; hyperactivity; caused birth defects and cancer in animal studies	Cake mix, jelly crystals, cereal, soft drinks, blackcurrant products	Pet foods, lipstick, blush and other cosmetics
Asthma; hyperactivity; hives; learning difficulties; light sensitivity; may affect liver, heart, reproduction, thyroid, stomach; suspected carcinogen	Canned fruit cocktail, cookies, crackers, glace cherries, canned red cherries, maraschino cherries, sausage casings	Pet foods, toothpaste, dental disclosing tablets, blush, medications
Asthma; hyperactivity; allergic reactions; hay fever; hives; caution advised if aspirin sensitive; adverse reproductive effects in animals; suspected carcinogen	Cake mix, jelly crystals, cereals, custards, jams, chocolate cakes and crackers, candy, bakery products	Pet foods, cosmetics, lipstick, shampoo, medications

Names	Function	Code	
FD&C Red No. 40 Aluminum Lake (may contain aluminum)	Coloring	☹	
FD&C Yellow No. 5 (tartrazine; synthetic; coal tar dye; from phenylhydrazine-4-sulfonic acid and dioxosuccinic acid; banned in foods in some countries; on the NIH HSDB)	Coloring (lemon yellow to orange)	☹	
FD&C Yellow No. 5 Calcium Lake (synthetic; coal tar dye)	Coloring	☹	
FD&C Yellow No. 6 (sunset yellow FCF; synthetic; azo dye; banned in foods in some countries)	Coloring (orange/yellow)	☹	
FD&C Yellow No. 6 Aluminum Lake (may contain aluminum)	Coloring	☹	
FD&C Yellow No. 6 Calcium Lake (synthetic; azo dye)	Coloring	☹	
Ferric chloride (on the NIH HSDB)	Flavoring	☹	

	Potential Effects	Possible Food Use	Other Uses
	See FD&C Red No. 40; see also aluminum	Candy, candy, decorating eggshells	Pet foods
	Dermatitis; concentration difficulties; depression; hay fever; learning difficulties; headache; hives; asthma; skin rash; behavioral problems; swelling of lips and tongue; hyperactivity; anaphylaxis; aggressive behavior; insomnia; confusion; NRC; caution advised if aspirin sensitive	Candy, canned or frozen corn, cheese crackers, soft drinks, mint sauce, mint jelly, fruit juice cordial, canned peas, marzipan, pickles, steak sauce, packet dessert topping, jams, cereal, packaged soups	Pet foods, toothpaste, shampoo, aftershave, cosmetics, wool and silk dye; pharmaceuticals
	See FD&C Yellow No. 5	Candy, candy, decorating eggshells	Pet foods
	Asthma; hives, hay fever; abdominal pain; eczema; hives; hyperactivity; caution advised if aspirin sensitive	Fruit juice cordial, marzipan, dry soup mix, cereal, candy, dry drink powder, canned fish	Pet foods, cosmetics, hair rinses
	See FD&C Yellow No. 6; see also aluminum	Candy, candy, decorating eggshells	Pet foods
	See FD&C Yellow No. 6	Candy, candy, decorating eggshells	Pet foods
	Corrosive; moderate toxicity if ingested; caused abnormal reproductive effects in animal studies; may destroy vitamin E	Various processed foods	Photography, pigments

Names	Function	Code	
Ferrous gluconate (iron bound to gluconic acid)	Color retention agent	☺?	
Ferrous lactate (may be derived from lactic acid and iron filings)	Coloring	☺?	
Ferrous sulfate (inorganic form of iron bound to sulfur; on the NIH HSDB)	Yeast food	☺?	
Ficin (enzyme found in the latex of fig trees; may be GE)	Food enzyme	☺	
Folic acid (folate; water-soluble 'B' group vitamin; synthetic; on the NIH HSDB)	Nutrient additive	☺	
Formaldehyde (gas derived from the oxidation of methyl alcohol; on the Canadian Hotlist; on the NIH HSDB)	Preservative	☹☹	
Formic acid (by-product of formaldehyde; on the NIH HSDB)	Preservative Flavoring Rubefacient	☹☹	

Potential Effects	Possible Food Use	Other Uses
Stomach upsets; caused tumors in animal studies; iron is potentially toxic in all forms	Ripe olives	
Caused tumors in animal studies; iron is potentially toxic in all forms	Black olives	
Constipation; nausea; destroys vitamin E; gastrointestinal, liver, kidney, cardiovascular and neurotoxicity	Bacterial cultures, flavoring in processed foods	Hair dye, cosmetics, medical treatment of anemia
Believed safe in food use at low levels; may cause skin, eye and mucous membrane irritation	Meat tenderizing preparations, to clot milk, beer, sausage casings, cheese	Protein digestant in cosmetics
Believed safe in food use; considered to have many beneficial health effects; adverse effects are rare	Enriched bread, pasta, rice, grain products	Shampoo, hair conditioner, pharmaceutical preparations
Eye, nose & throat irritation; coughing; nose bleeds; reproductive, respiratory, gastrointestinal, liver, skin, immuno and neurotoxicity; human carcinogen	De-foaming additives used in processing foods like jams, jellies, fruit juice, baked goods, candies, milk products	Mascara, soap, shampoo, bubble bath, nail polish, nail hardener, anti-aging cream, filler in vaccines
Cardiovascular, respiratory, gastrointestinal, kidney, liver and neurotoxicity; cancer in animal studies	Various processed foods	Silage (animal fodder), hair tonic, paint remover

Names	Function	Code	
Fructose (fruit sugar; may be from corn; produced commercially using enzymes; probably GE; on the NIH HSDB)	Sweetener Preservative	☺?	
Fumaric Acid (by fermentation of glucose or molasses by fungi; may be synthetic)	Buffer Antioxidant	☺☺	
Furcelleran (extract from the red seaweed *Furcellaria fastigiata* and processed as a gum)	Emulsifier Thickener Stabilizer	☺	.
Furfural (artificial ant oil; synthetic)	Flavoring Solvent	☹☹	
Furfuryl alcohol (synthetic; derived from furfural)	Flavoring	☹	
Gelatin (from pigskins, cowhides, bones; of ANIMAL origin; on the NIH HSDB)	Stabilizer Thickener	☺	
Gellan gum (made by fermentation of a carbohydrate with the bacteria *Pseudomonas elodea*)	Stabilizer Thickener	☺	

Potential Effects	Possible Food Use	Other Uses
Believed safe in food use at low levels; excess may increase risk of tooth decay, obesity, gout, kidney stones, colon cancer	High fructose corn syrup (HFCS) used in processed foods like soft drinks, ice cream, jam, ketchup, candy	Moisturizer, skin cleanser
Believed safe in food use	Candy, baked goods, desserts, dietary supplements	Cosmetics
Believed safe in food use; on a list of additives to be studied for mutagenic, reproductive, teratogenic and sub-acute effects	Ice cream, jams, desserts, diabetic products	Toothpaste
Persistent headache; eye problems; respiratory, skin, kidney, gastrointestinal, liver and neurotoxicity; suspected carcinogen and mutagen	Processed foods like beverages, ice cream, candy, baked goods, syrups, spirits	Insecticide, fungicide
Respiratory and neurotoxicity; highly toxic when concentrated	Processed foods like beverages, ice cream, candy, baked goods	
May contain sulfur dioxide and/or MSG which can have adverse effects on some people	Mustard pickles, meat loaf, relishes, cottage cheese, sausage casings, ice cream	Nail strengthener, protein shampoo, body soap, filler in vaccines
Believed safe in food use at low levels; excess can cause diarrhea; eye and skin irritation	Processed foods	

Names	Function	Code	
Geraniol and geranyl compounds (geraniol derived from palmerosa oil or synthetically from pinene; geraniol is on the NIH HSDB)	Flavoring Additive	☺?	
Ghatti gum (extract from a plant native to India and Sri Lanka)	Emulsifier Stabilizer	☺	
Glucanase (enzyme from fungi; probably GE)	Food enzyme	☺	
Glucoamylase (derived from enzymes from mold; may be GE)	Food enzyme	☺☺	
Gluconic acid (made synthetically from corn; probably GE)	Anti-caking agent Sequestrant	☺	
Glucono delta lactone (made from the oxidation of glucose; may be GE)	Buffer	☺	
Glucose isomerase (produced from various strains of bacteria; probably GE)	Food enzyme	☺	
Glycerin (glycerol; synthetic; by-product of soap manufacture; may be of ANIMAL origin; on the NIH HSDB)	Humectant Solvent	☺	

Potential Effects	Possible Food Use	Other Uses
Allergic reactions; mucous membrane irritation; contact dermatitis; moderately toxic if ingested	Processed foods like beverages, ice cream, candy, baked goods, chewing gum	Perfume, soap, shampoo, cosmetics, cigarettes
Believed safe in food use at low levels; may cause allergic reactions in some	Processed foods, alcoholic beverages	
Believed safe in food use	Unstandardized bakery products, beer, stout	
Believed safe in food use	Bread, flour, instant cereals, chocolate syrup, beer, ale	
Believed safe in food use	Unstandardized foods, dietary supplements	Metal cleaners
Believed safe in food use at low levels; excess can cause diarrhea	Cottage cheese, meat processing, canned vegetables, brewing beer	Cleaning agents
Believed safe in food use	Used to produce high-fructose syrups for making candy and soft drinks	
Believed safe in foods at low levels; excess can cause headache; mental confusion; may affect heart, reproduction, stomach, blood sugar level	Candy, dried fruit, low calorie foods, marshmallows, baked goods, chewing gum	Soap, toothpaste, perfumes, hand cream, tobacco, mouthwash, protective cream, filler in vaccines

Names	Function	Code	
Glycerol ester of wood rosin (made from wood rosin and food grade glycerol; may be of ANIMAL origin)	Emulsifier Stabilizer	☺	
Glyceryl diacetate	Carrier or extraction solvent	☺	
Glyceryl monostearate	Emulsifier Dispersant	☺	
Glyceryl triacetate (triacetin; from acetic acid and glycerin; on the NIH HSDB)	Carrier or extraction solvent Fixative	☺	
Glyceryl tributyrate (tributyrin; from butyric acid and glycerin)	Carrier or extraction solvent Flavoring	☺?	
Glycine (nonessential amino acid; may be synthetic; may be of ANIMAL origin; on the NIH HSDB)	Sequestrant Texturiser	☺?	
Gold (naturally occurring metal)	Coloring (metallic)	☺	
Guar Gum (obtained from the seeds of a tree in India)	Thickener Stabilizer	☺	
Gum arabic (acacia gum)	Thickener Emulsifier	☺?	

Potential Effects	Possible Food Use	Other Uses
See glycerol	Citrus-flavored beverages, chewing gum base	Liquid adhesive
See glyceryl triacetate	See glyceryl triacetate	
Believed safe in food use; high dose injections proved fatal to mice	Noodles, pasta products, shortenings	Hair conditioner, hand lotion, baby cream, mascara
Believed safe in food use; eye irritation; high dose injections were fatal to rats	Preparation of flavorings used in processed foods	Toothpaste, hair dye, cigarette filters, perfume
Believed safe in food use; moderately toxic when ingested	Preparation of flavorings used in processed foods	
Believed safe in food use at low levels; excess can have adverse health effects including fatigue	Dietary supplements, processed foods containing saccharin to mask the aftertaste	Cosmetics, shampoo, antacid
Believed safe in food use; rare allergic reactions; neurotoxicity	External decoration on chocolate confections, alcoholic beverages	Cosmetics
Believed safe in food use at low levels; abdominal cramps; nausea; flatulence; diarrhea from excess; asthma and hay fever when in its dry form	Baked goods, jam, cereals, jellies, cheese spreads, beverages, infant foods, toppings	Tablet binding agent, cosmetics, pet foods, diet aids (caution recommended)
See acacia gum	See acacia gum	See acacia gum

Names	Function	Code	
Gum benzoin (extract from trees native to parts of SE Asia)	Flavoring Glazing and polishing agent	☺	
Gum furcelleran (furcelleran)	Emulsifier Thickener Stabilizer	☺	
Gum ghatti (ghatti gum)	Emulsifier Stabilizer	☺	
Gum guaiac (gum guaiacum; extract from *Guaiacum officinale*)	Antioxidant Flavoring	☺	
Heliotropin (piperonal; purple diazo dye)	Flavoring Additive	☻?	
Helium (from natural gas)	Propellant Packaging gas	☺	
Hemicellulase (xylanase; enzyme from fungi or bacteria; probably GE)	Food enzyme	☺	
Heptylparaben (synthetic)	Preservative	☹	
Hexane (n-hexane; from gasoline, toluene, benzene or xylene; on the NIH HSDB)	Carrier or extraction solvent	☹☹	
Hexylresorcinol (4-hexylresorcinol; see also resorcinol in section 2)	Color stabilizer Preservative	☹	

Potential Effects	Possible Food Use	Other Uses
Believed safe in food use; suspected mutagen	Processed foods like beverages, ice cream, candy, baked goods, candy	Cosmetic creams, skin protectant
See furcelleran	See furcelleran	See furcelleran
See ghatti gum	See ghatti gum	
Believed safe in food use at low levels; may cause allergic reactions in some	Fats and oils, lard, shortening, alcoholic beverages	Cosmetic creams and lotions
Allergic reactions; skin irritation; CNS depression on ingestion of large amounts	Cherry and vanilla flavors in processed foods	Perfume, soap
Believed safe in food use; respiratory toxicity	Foods packaged in pressurized containers	Arc welding, inflating balloons
Believed safe in food use	Liquid coffee concentrate, vinegar manufacture	
See parabens in section 2	Malt beverages, fruit-based beverages	
Respiratory, reproductive, developmental and neurotoxicity; suspected teratogen	Spice extracts, extracting vegetable fats and oils	Laundry starch, rubber cement, furniture polish, pharmaceuticals
Can cause bowel, liver and heart damage, and severe gastrointestinal irritation	Uncooked crustacea	Mouthwash, sunburn cream, antiseptic

Names	Function	Code	
High fructose corn syrup (HFCS; fructose combined with dextrose; probably GE)	Sweetener	☺?	
Hydrazine (from chloramine, ammonia and sodium hydroxide; on the Canadian Hotlist)	Solvent Reducing agent	☹	
Hydrochloric acid (HCl; strong mineral acid; mostly as a byproduct from chlorination processes; on the NIH HSDB)	Buffer Starch modifying agent	☺?	
Hydrogen peroxide (made from barium peroxide and diluted phosphoric acid; on the Canadian Hotlist; on the NIH HSDB)	Preservative Bleaching agent Maturing agent	☺?	
Hydrogenated starch hydrolysates (synthetic; derived from corn syrup; probably GE)	Sweetener	☺	

Potential Effects	Possible Food Use	Other Uses
See fructose	See fructose	
Toxic if inhaled, ingested or absorbed through the skin; kidney, cardiovascular, immuno and neurotoxicity; recognized carcinogen; suspected teratogen; very toxic to aquatic organisms	Steam that comes into contact with foods (zero residue permitted)	Cosmetics, corrosion inhibitor, pharmaceuticals
Fume inhalation causes choking and inflammation of respiratory tract; liver, respiratory, gastrointestinal, musculoskeletal and immunotoxicity	Cottage cheese, cream cheese, infant formula, modified food starch	Hair bleach, tile cleaner, solvent, toilet bowl cleaner
Believed safe in cosmetics as a preservative; corrosive to skin, eyes & respiratory tract when undiluted; may cause allergic reactions, headache; nausea; toxic to aquatic organisms	Swiss cheese, cheddar cheese, butter, milk	Cosmetics, mouthwash, toothpaste, disinfectants, medicinal antiseptic and germicide
Believed safe in food use; may cause stomach upsets	Unstandardized foods	Toothpaste

Names	Function	Code	
Hydrogenated vegetable oil (contains MSG; probably GE)	Flavor enhancer	☹	
Hydrolyzed protein (of ANIMAL origin (see pepsin, trypsin); contains MSG)	Flavoring Flavor enhancer	☺?	
Hydrolyzed vegetable protein (HVP; contains MSG; may be of ANIMAL origin (see pepsin, trypsin); may be GE)	Flavor enhancer Antistatic agent	☺?	
Hydroxylated lecithin	Antioxidant Emulsifier	☺☺	
Hydroxypropyl cellulose (synthetic ether of cellulose; may be GE)	Thickener Emulsifier	☺	
Hydroxypropyl methylcellulose (synthetic; from cellulose; may be GE)	Thickener Emulsifier	☺	

Potential Effects	Possible Food Use	Other Uses
Hydrogenation creates trans-fatty acids which can increase risk of high blood pressure, atherosclerosis, cancers, obesity, diabetes mellitus type 2, Alzheimer's disease and heart disease	Baked goods, cakes, cookies, instant soups, sauces, beef stew, corn chips, salad dressing, doughnuts, easy-to-spread butter, margarine	Eye shadow, hair products, cleansing lotion
May cause contamination with carcinogenic nitrosamines; see MSG	Soups, stews, sauces	Animal feed, cosmetics, shampoo, hair treatments
Concerns associated with HVP include decreased body weight, organ atrophy, behavioral over-activity, brain and nervous system damage, bladder and bowel incontinence	Soups, stews, sauces, baby foods	Hair care products
Believed safe in food use	Chocolate and cocoa products, ice cream, margarine	Skin care products
Believed safe in food use; may cause allergic reactions	Low fat cream, UHT cream	Antiperspirant, hand gel, tobacco
Believed safe in food use; mild eye and skin irritation; allergic reactions	Candy, infant formula, icing, topping, ice cream, pickles, soup, dried mixed fruit	Cosmetics, bubble bath, tanning lotion, shampoo

Names	Function	Code	
Invert sugar (equal parts of glucose and fructose; probably GE)	Sweetener	☺	
Invertase (enzyme from brewer's yeast; may be GE)	Food enzyme	☺☺	
Ionone (synthetic)	Flavoring	☺?	
Iron oxide (rust; synthetic oxides of iron; banned in foods in some countries)	Coloring (red/brown/ black/ orange/yellow)	☺?	
Isoamyl acetate (synthetic)	Flavoring	☹	
Isoascorbic acid (erythorbic acid)	Antioxidant Preservative	☺	
Isobutane (from petroleum or natural gas; on the NIH HSDB)	Propellant	☺?	
Isobutyl alcohol (isobutanol; from propylene; on the NIH HSDB)	Solvent	☹	
Isomalt (produced from sugar; may be enhanced with acesulfame potassium)	Sweetener Humectant	☺?	

Potential Effects	Possible Food Use	Other Uses
Believed safe in food use at low levels; can contribute to dental caries	Candy, brewing industry	
Believed safe in food use	Flour, bread, yogurt, flavored milk, soft-centered confections	
Caused adverse effects in animal studies; may cause allergic reactions	Processed foods	Perfume
Iron is potentially toxic in all forms; excess can lead to increased risk of numerous health conditions	Salmon and shrimp paste or spread, cake and dessert mixes	Pet foods, dying egg shells, face powder, eye makeup
Can cause headaches, fatigue, mucous membrane irritation; neurotoxicity	Processed foods like beverages, ice cream, candy, baked goods	Perfume
See erythorbic acid	See erythorbic acid	See erythorbic acid
See butane	Non-stick cooking spray	Cosmetic spray, refrigeration
Toxic by inhalation; skin and mucous membrane irritation; dermatitis; neurotoxicity	Synthetic fruit flavorings used in processed foods	Shampoo, paint stripper, perfume, cleaning agents
Believed safe in food use at low levels; excess may cause gastrointestinal upsets	Ice cream, jams, baked goods	Cosmetics

Names	Function	Code	
Isopropanol (isopropyl alcohol)	Solvent Antifoaming agent	☹	
Isopropyl alcohol (isopropanol; derived from petroleum; on the NIH HSDB)	Solvent Antifoaming agent	☹	
Isopropyl citrate (synthetic)	Antioxidant Sequestrant	☺	
Karaya gum (sterculia gum; exudate of a tree found in India)	Thickener Stabilizer	😐?	
Kola nut extract (extract from the seeds of cola trees; contains caffeine)	Flavoring	😐?	
Konjac, konjac flour (derived from the tubers of a plant grown in Japan; banned in some countries)	Emulsifier Thickener	😐?	
Lactic acid (may be from whey, cornstarch, potatoes or molasses; may be synthetic; may be GE; may be of ANIMAL origin; on the NIH HSDB)	Preservative Acidulant	☺	
Lactitol (derived from milk sugar (lactose); of ANIMAL origin; may be GE)	Sweetener Flavoring	☺☺	

Potential Effects	Possible Food Use	Other Uses
See isopropyl alcohol	See isopropyl alcohol	See isopropyl alcohol
Skin irritation; respiratory, gastrointestinal, liver, kidney, developmental and neurotoxicity; suspected teratogen	Spice extracts, food flavorings	Perfume, hair color rinse, body lotion, shampoo, cleansing cream
See citrates	Salad oils, oleomargarine	
Asthma; hives; hay fever; dermatitis; reduces nutrient intake; gastric irritation	Ice cream, baked goods, sweets, gumdrops, frozen dairy desserts	Hair spray, hand lotion, toothpaste
See caffeine	Processed foods like beverages, ice cream, candy, baked goods	"Organic" cosmetics
Choking hazard in dry form; diarrhea; abdominal pain; stomach problems; nutrient disruption	Soups, gravy, jam, bread, mayonnaise, candy	
Believed safe in foods; contact can cause stinging of the skin in sensitive people; not recommended for babies under 3 months	Infant formula, cheese, salad dressing, relish, candy, soft drinks, tartare sauce, margarine	Cosmetics, skin fresheners, hair conditioner, body wash, cigarettes
Believed safe in food use	Baked goods, chewing gum	

Names	Function	Code	
Lactose (milk sugar from whey; may be synthetic; may be of ANIMAL origin; may be GE)	Nutrient additive Humectant	☺	
Larch gum (arabinogalactin)	Thickener Stabilizer	☺?	
Lecithin (residue from making soybean oil; may be GE; on the NIH HSDB)	Antioxidant Emulsifier Emollient	☺	
Lecithin citrate (may be GE)	Emulsifier	☺	
Lemon oil (extract from lemon peel; on the NIH HSDB)	Flavoring Fragrance	☺?	
Leucine (L-leucine & DL-leucine; essential amino acid; may be of ANIMAL origin; may be GE)	Flavor enhancer	☺	
Levulose (fructose; may be GE)	Sweetener	☺?	
Licorice and licorice oils (from the herb *Glycyrrhiza glabra*)	Flavoring	☺?	
Lime oil (from the fruit of a tropical tree)	Flavoring	☺	

Potential Effects	Possible Food Use	Other Uses
Regarded as safe in food use at low levels; excess can cause adverse health effects like tooth decay, diarrhea, irritable bowel syndrome, intestinal cramp	Used to sour milk, infant formula	Eye drops, tablet preparation, anti-wrinkle treatment
See arabinogalactin	See arabinogalactin	See arabinogalactin
Believed safe in food use; people with allergy to soy may wish to avoid	Chocolate, dried milk, margarine, cake mix, candy	Lipstick, hand cream, mascara, pharmaceuticals
See lecithin and citrates	See lecithin	
Allergic reactions; photoallergy	Processed foods like beverages, ice cream, candy, baked goods	Perfume, aftershave, hair conditioner
Has beneficial health effects; excess may interfere with other substances in the body	Tabletop sweetener	
See fructose	See fructose	
Intestinal upset, headache, asthma, contact dermatitis	Processed foods like beverages, ice cream, candy, baked goods, chewing gum	Hair conditioner, skin moisturizer, tobacco
Believed safe in food use; may cause a sensitivity to light when used on the skin	Processed foods like beverages, ice cream, candy, baked goods, chewing gum	Perfume, soap, bath preparations (bubbles, bathmilk, oils)

Names	Function	Code
Limonene (d-limonene; from mandarin peel oil; on the NIH HSDB)	Flavoring Fragrance	☹
Linalool (linalyl alcohol; extract from oils of lavender, bergamot & coriander; on the NIH HSDB)	Flavoring Additive	☺?
Linden extract (from flowers of the Linden tree)	Flavoring Fragrance	☺☺
Lipase (may be from fungi, castor beans or of ANIMAL origin; probably GE)	Food enzyme	☺
Locust bean gum (carob bean gum; carob)	Thickener Emulsifier	☺☺
Lysine (may be from casein, fibrin or blood; may be synthetic; may be of ANIMAL origin; may be GE; on the NIH HSDB)	Nutrient additive	☺☺
Lysozyme (enzyme from egg white; of ANIMAL origin; may be GE)	Food enzyme	☺☺
Magnesium aluminum silicate (Fuller's Earth)	Dusting agent Thickener	☺?

Potential Effects	Possible Food Use	Other Uses
Sensitization, skin irritation, has caused weight loss and tumors in animal studies; animal carcinogen; may bio-accumulate in fish and aquatic organisms	Processed foods like beverages, ice cream, candy, baked goods, chewing gum	Perfume, soap, manufacture of resins
Allergic reactions; facial psoriasis; mildly toxic by ingestion; skin and eye irritation; may effect the liver	Chocolate, lemon and blueberry flavorings in processed foods	Perfumed soap, aftershave, hand lotion, hairspray, anti-wrinkle treatment
Believed to have beneficial health effects	Raspberry & vermouth flavors used in foods	Moisturizer, hair care products
Believed safe in food use	Liquid and dried egg whites, bread, flour, edible fats and oils, cheese manufacture	Bleach, septic tank treatment
Believed safe in food use; may lower cholesterol levels	Infant formula, ice cream, pickles, icings, toppings, chutney, cheese, candy	Depilatories, animal feed, detergent, adhesives
Believed safe in food use; considered to have beneficial health effects	Wheat-based foods, specialty breads	Shampoo, skin cleanser, hair conditioner, animal feed
Believed safe in food use	Cheese manufacture	Skin conditioner
Caused kidney damage when ingested by dogs; see aluminum	Chewing gum	Cosmetics

Names	Function	Code	
Magnesium carbonate (synthetic; from magnesium sulfate and sodium carbonate; on the NIH HSDB)	Anti-caking agent	☺	
Magnesium chloride (synthetic; from hydrochloric acid and magnesium oxide/hydroxide; on the NIH HSDB)	Firming agent Buffer	☺	
Magnesium citrate (magnesium bound to citric acid; may be corn-based; may be GE)	Buffer	☺	
Magnesium fumarate (magnesium bound to fumaric acid; may be corn-based; may be GE)	Acidifier	☺	
Magnesium gluconate (magnesium bound to gluconic acid)	Buffer	☺	
Magnesium hydroxide (from magnesium chloride and sodium hydroxide or precipitation of seawater)	Buffer	☺	
Magnesium oxide (from magnesite ores; magnesium bound to oxide; on the NIH HSDB)	Anti-caking agent Firming agent	☺?	
Magnesium phosphate (magnesium bound to phosphorus)	Anti-caking agent Nutrient additive	☺	

Potential Effects	Possible Food Use	Other Uses
Believed safe in food use at low levels; excess may have a laxative effect	Sour cream, ice cream, canned peas, table salt, mineral water	Foundation, face powder, mascara
Believed safe in food use at low levels; excess may have a laxative effect; caution advised if kidney function is impaired	Infant formula, salt substitute, non-alcoholic beverages	Shampoo, facial cleanser
See citrates; caution advised if kidney function is impaired	Soft drinks	Products designed to add body or volume to hair
Believed safe in food use; readily absorbed orally; caution advised if kidney function is impaired	Unstandardized foods	
Believed safe in food use; caution advised if kidney function is impaired	Soda water	
Believed safe in food use at low levels; caution advised if kidney function is impaired	Manufacture of some caramels, canned peas, cheese manufacture	Dentifrices, skin cream
Caution advised if kidney function is impaired; excess may cause diarrhea; tumors in animal studies	Frozen dairy products, canned peas, butter	Hair bleach, bath products, animal feed, cosmetics
Believed safe in food use; caution advised if kidney function is impaired	Dried milk, milk powder, dietary supplements	

Names	Function	Code	
Magnesium silicate (magnesium bound to silica; on the NIH HSDB)	Anti-caking agent Bleaching agent	☺	
Magnesium stearate (from magnesium sulfate and sodium stearate; on the NIH HSDB)	Anti-caking agent Release agent Emulsifier	☺?	
Magnesium sulfate (magnesium bound to sulfur; Epsom salts is hydrated form; on the NIH HSDB)	Firming agent Nutrient additive	☺	
Malic acid (from be from natural sources or synthetic from benzene; on the NIH HSDB)	Buffer Antioxidant	☺	
Mallow extract (extract from the herb *Malva sylvestris*)	Coloring (dark red)	☺☺	
Maltitol, maltitol syrup (from maltose (malt sugar); may be GE)	Sweetener Stabilizer	☺?	
Maltodextrin (maltol and dextrin; usually from corn starch; probably GE)	Flavor enhancer	☺	

Potential Effects	Possible Food Use	Other Uses
Believed safe in food use at low levels; kidney stones; caution advised if kidney function is impaired	Vanilla powder, table salt, animal and vegetable oils	Shampoo, mascara, paints, varnishes
Slightly toxic by ingestion; caution advised if kidney function is impaired; safety is being reviewed	Icing sugar, salt, garlic salt, onion salt	Cosmetics, baby powder, bar soap, tablets
Excess may have a laxative effect; caution advised if kidney function is impaired	Infant formula as a nutrient additive, brewing beer	Cosmetic lotions, body wash, hair conditioner
Believed safe in food use; skin & mucous membrane irritation; may aggravate herpes simplex symptoms	Sweetened coconut, canned oxtail soup, low calorie soft drinks, wines	Nail polish, hair conditioner, pet shampoo
Believed safe in food use; thought to have anti-inflammatory properties	Natural coloring in foods, source of pectin	Body wash
Caused benign & malignant tumors and breast cancer in animal studies; laxative effect with excess	Low calorie foods, dried fruit, candy	Moisturizer
Believed safe in foods at low levels; excess may elevate blood sugar and insulin levels and increase risk of diabetes mellitus	Chocolate, candy	Hair conditioner, mascara

Names	Function	Code	
Maltose (malt sugar; may be soy, corn or wheat-based; probably GE)	Sweetener Humectant	☺?	
Manganese sulfate (from hydroquinone production or manganous hydroxide and sulfuric acid; on the NIH HSDB)	Nutrient additive	☺?	
Mannitol (prepared from seaweed)	Sweetener Humectant	☹	
Menthol (natural or synthetically made from thymol)	Flavoring	☺	
Methanol (methyl alcohol)	Carrier or extraction solvent	☹	
Methionine (essential amino acid; may be GE)	Nutrient additive	☺	
Methyl acetate (synthetic; may be from methanol & acetic acid; on the NIH HSDB)	Flavoring Solvent	☹	

Potential Effects	Possible Food Use	Other Uses
May contribute to tooth decay; caused tumors in animal studies	Processed foods	Cosmetics
Believed safe in food use; those with liver cirrhosis should avoid; neurotoxicity; lethal if injected into mice	Dietary supplements	Red hair dye, lawn fertilizer, animal feeds, glass making
Hypersensitivity reactions; nausea; vomiting; diarrhea; hives; NRC and diabetics; kidney dysfunction; gastric irritation; anaphylaxis	Carbohydrate-modified foods or low calorie foods, chewing gum, sweets, jams, jellies	Hand cream, hair grooming products
Believed safe in food use at low levels; toxic when concentrated	Processed foods like beverages, ice cream, candy, baked goods	Mouthwash, perfumes, cigarettes
See methyl alcohol	See methyl alcohol	See methyl alcohol
Believed safe in foods at low levels; excess may have adverse effects on body organs; people with schizophrenia should avoid	Should not be used in baby foods	Hair conditioner, shampoo, hand cleaner
Can cause chafing and cracking of the skin; respiratory & neurotoxicity	Processed foods like beverages, ice cream, candy, baked goods	Perfume, paint remover, resins and oils

Names	Function	Code	
Methyl alcohol (methanol; from carbon monoxide and hydrogen; on the Canadian Hotlist; on the NIH HSDB)	Carrier or extraction solvent	☹	
Methyl anthranilate (synthetic, from coal tar; on the NIH HSDB)	Flavoring Fragrance	☺?	
Methyl cellulose (may be from wood pulp or chemical cotton; may be GE; on the NIH HSDB)	Thickener Stabilizer	☺	
Methylene chloride (dichloromethane; on the Canadian Hotlist; banned in cosmetics in the EU and USA; on the NIH HSDB)	Carrier or extraction solvent	☹☹	
Methyl ethyl cellulose (from wood pulp or chemical cotton)	Emulsifier Aerating agent	☺?	
Methyl ethyl ketone (MEK; 2-butanone; synthetic; usually from butyl alcohol; on the NIH HSDB)	Carrier or extraction solvent	☹	

Potential Effects	Possible Food Use	Other Uses
Dermatitis; kidney, liver, developmental, respiratory, gastrointestinal and neurotoxicity	Extraction of hops and spices, component of aspartame, alcoholic beverages	Deodorant, shampoo, household cleaners
Skin irritation; see coal tar	Processed foods like beverages, ice cream, candy, baked goods	Perfume, suntan lotion, cigarettes
Believed safe in food use at low levels; laxative effect with excess	Infant formula, toppings, ice cream, pickles, chutney, candy, imitation fruit, soup	Cosmetics, hand cream and lotion, sun cream, slimming aids
Cardiovascular, respiratory, reproductive, endocrine, gastrointestinal, kidney, liver and neurotoxicity; skin irritation; carcinogen; environmental hazard	Decaffeinated roasted coffee, decaffeinated instant coffee, spice extracts, decaffeinated instant tea, decaffeinated tea leaves	Nail polish, hair spray, furniture polish, tablet coatings, disinfectants
See sodium carboxymethyl cellulose	Unstandardized foods, vegetable-fat whipped topping	
Cardiovascular, respiratory, gastrointestinal, liver, kidney, reproductive, developmental and neurotoxicity	Spice extracts, vegetable oil, processed foods	Perfumes, nail polish, shampoo, paint thinner, shoe polish, car cleaner & polish

Names	Function	Code
Methyl isobutyl ketone (MIBK; synthetic; on the NIH HSDB)	Flavoring Solvent	☹☹
Methylparaben (methyl-p-hydroxybenzoate; on the NIH HSDB)	Preservative	☹
Methyl-p-hydroxy benzoate (methylparaben)	Preservative	☹
Methyl salicylate (oil of wintergreen; may be synthetic; on the Canadian Hotlist; on the NIH HSDB)	Flavoring Disinfectant	☹
Microcrystalline cellulose (cellulose microcrystalline)	Thickener Stabilizer Filler	☺
Mineral oil (derived from petroleum)	Glazing and polishing agent Release agent	☹
Modified food starch (may be GE)	Thickener Binder	☹

Potential Effects	Possible Food Use	Other Uses
Hazardous by ingestion or inhalation; kidney, liver, gastrointestinal, respiratory and neurotoxicity; birth defects; dermatitis	Synthetic fruit flavoring in processed foods like ice cream, ices, candy, baked goods	Perfume, solvent for cellulose and lacquer, paint, varnish
See parabens in section 2	Preserves, jelly	Cosmetics, bubble bath
See methylparaben	See methylparaben	See methylparaben
Strong irritant to the skin and mucous membranes; blood, liver, reproductive, respiratory & neurotoxicity; suspected teratogen; toxic to aquatic organisms	Processed foods like beverages, ice cream, candy, baked goods	Toothpaste, mouthwash, sunburn treatment lotion, detergents, cigarettes, toilet bowl cleaner
See cellulose microcrystalline	See cellulose microcrystalline	See cellulose microcrystalline
Inhalation causes birth defects; testicular tumors in the fetus; may inhibit proper skin function; avoid during pregnancy	Candy, fresh fruits and vegetables, bakery products	Capsules and tablets, baby creams & lotions, lipstick, hand cleaner
See starch, food, modified	See starch, food, modified	

Names	Function	Code	
Mono- and diglycerides (may be synthetic; esters of glycerol and fatty acids; may be from soy, corn or peanuts; probably GE)	Emulsifier Stabilizer Texturiser	☺	
Monoisopropyl citrate	Preservative	☺	
Monopotassium glutamate (synthetic; may be GE)	Flavor enhancer	☹	
Monosodium glutamate (MSG; monosodium salt of glutamic acid; probably GE)	Flavor enhancer	☹	
Monosodium salts of phosphorylated mono- and diglycerides	Emulsifier	☺	
Morpholine (from diethanolamine or ethylene oxide and ammonia; on the Canadian Hotlist; on the NIH HSDB)	Solvent Emulsifier	☹☹	
MSG (monosodium glutamate)	Flavor enhancer	☹	

Potential Effects	Possible Food Use	Other Uses
Believed safe in food use; diglycerides are under investigation by the FDA for possible teratogenic, reproductive, mutagenic and sub-acute effects	Bakery products, ice cream, oleomargarine, beverages, chocolate, candy	Cosmetic creams
See citrates	Fats and oils, margarine, meats, sausage, lard	Food packaging materials
See monosodium glutamate	See monosodium glutamate	
Bronchospasm; irritability; heart palpitations; nausea; abdominal discomfort; fibromyalgia; blurred vision; asthma; vertigo; headache; depression; migraine; sight impairment; NRC; caution advised if aspirin sensitive	May be found in dried or instant soup, flavored noodles, textured protein, malt extract, yeast extract, soy sauce, gelatin, flavorings (chicken, beef, pork, smoke)	Hidden sources of MSG including soap, cosmetics, shampoo, hair conditioner, most live virus vaccines, pet foods
See mono- and diglycerides	Non-stick-spray	
Respiratory, kidney, liver, gastrointestinal, skin, and neurotoxicity; skin, mucous membrane & eye damage	Coating on fresh fruits and vegetables for shine	Shampoo, dyes, cosmetic creams, metal polish, car polish and wax
See monosodium glutamate	See monosodium glutamate	See monosodium glutamate

Names	Function	Code	
Musk (dried secretion from a deer; of ANIMAL origin)	Flavoring Fragrance	☺	
Musk ambrette (of ANIMAL origin; banned from cosmetics in the EU; on the Canadian Hotlist)	Flavoring Fixative Fragrance	☹	
Myristic acid (long-chain saturated fatty acid; may be of ANIMAL origin; on the NIH HSDB)	Flavoring Emulsifier	☺?	
Natamycin (pimaricin; fungicide from *Streptomyces natalensis*; probably GE)	Preservative	☹	
Neotame (similar to aspartame; 7000 to 13,000 times sweeter than sugar; contains aspartic acid, phenylalanine and a methyl ester; may be GE)	Sweetener Flavor enhancer	☹	
Niacin (nicotinic acid, acid form of vitamin B3; synthetic; may be GE; on the NIH HSDB)	Nutrient additive	☺	

Potential Effects	Possible Food Use	Other Uses
Generally safe and non-toxic; can cause allergic reactions in some people	Processed foods like beverages, ice cream, candy, baked goods	Perfume, body lotion, aftershave
Neurotoxic; photosensitivity; contact dermatitis; serious brain damage in animals	Processed foods like beverages, ice cream, candy, baked goods	Perfume, soap, aftershave lotion, dentifrices, detergents
Believed safe in food use at low levels; may increase the risk of atherosclerosis; can cause skin irritation; caused mutations in laboratory animals	Processed foods like beverages, ice cream, candy, baked goods	Shampoo, skin creams, shaving cream, cigarettes
Moderately toxic by ingestion; nausea; vomiting; diarrhea; anorexia; mild skin irritation	Cured or processed meats, cheese rind	Drug used to treat fungal infections of the eyes and eyelids
Some renowned and respected scientists believe this synthetic compound to be toxic and capable of causing cancer and other adverse health effects	See aspartame	
Believed safe in food use; considered to have many beneficial health effects; in excess of 100mg/day may (rarely) cause side effects	Breakfast cereals, baby cereals, enriched flours, dietary supplements	Anti-aging products, hair conditioner

Names	Function	Code	
Niacinamide (form of vitamin B3; synthetic)	Nutrient additive	☺☺	
Nicotinic acid (niacin)	Nutrient additive	☺	
Nisin (crystals from the bacteria *Streptococcus lactis*; probably GE)	Preservative Anti-microbial	☺?	
Nitrogen (natural gas)	Propellant Packing gas	☺☺	
Nitropropane (1-nitropropane; from propane and nitric acid)	Carrier or extraction solvent	☹	
Nitrosyl chloride	Bleaching agent	☺?	
Nitrous oxide (laughing gas; from ammonium nitrate; on the NIH HSDB)	Propellant	☺	
Nutrasweet	Sweetener Flavor enhancer	☹	
Oat flour (ground oats with bran removed; contains gluten)	Thickener	☺?	

Potential Effects	Possible Food Use	Other Uses
Believed safe in food use at low levels	Dietary supplements	Shampoo, hand cleaner, makeup
See niacin	See niacin	See niacin
The European Parliament said in 2003 that it should not be used as it could cause antibiotic resistance in humans	Processed cheese, canned vegetables and fruit, semolina and tapioca puddings	Cosmetics
Believed safe in food use	Freezing and vacuum packing of foods	Preservative in cosmetics
Cardiovascular, respiratory, developmental, liver, gastrointestinal, reproductive and neurotoxicity	Vegetable fats and oils	Vinyl resin, dyes, synthetic rubber, waxes, lacquer, gasoline
Mucous membrane, skin and eye irritation; bleeding and pulmonary edema if inhaled	Cereal flour	
Believed safe in food use; developmental, reproductive & neurotoxicity	Flour (bleached), whipped cream	Whipped cosmetic cream
See aspartame	See aspartame	See aspartame
People with celiac disease should avoid; exacerbation of the symptoms of autism	Cereals, bread	Body wash, baby lotion, shave gel, hair conditioner

Names	Function	Code
Oat gum (extract from oats; contains gluten)	Stabilizer Thickener Antioxidant	☺?
Oatmeal (ground oats; contains gluten)	Thickener	☺?
Octafluorocyclobutane (used alone or combined with carbon dioxide or nitrous oxide)	Propellant Aerating agent	☺
Octyl gallate (synthetic; salt of gallic acid)	Antioxidant	☺?
Olestra (synthetic; not absorbed by the body; devoid of calories)	Fat substitute	☹
Orange oil (from the fresh peel of the sweet orange; on the NIH HSDB)	Flavoring Fragrance	☺
Oxystearin (glycerides of stearic acid and others; may be from corn; may be GE)	Crystallization inhibitor	☺?

Potential Effects	Possible Food Use	Other Uses
Allergic reactions such as bloating and diarrhea; people with celiac disease should avoid; exacerbation of the symptoms of autism	Cream cheese, cheese spread, candy, butter	Cosmetics
See oat flour	Cereals, bread	Face masks, moisturizer
Believed safe in foods when used alone; cardiovascular toxicity	Foamed or sprayed food products	
Mildly toxic by ingestion; allergic reactions; gastric irritation; caution advised if aspirin sensitive	Edible fats and oils, reduced fat spread, margarine	
Intestinal cramp; flatulence; diarrhea; obesity; may prevent the absorption of fat-soluble vitamins	French fries, crackers, baked desserts	
Allergic reactions if hypersensitive; severe reactions may occur to concentrated oil of orange	Processed foods like beverages, ice cream, candy, baked goods, chewing gum	Perfume, soap, skin lotion, cologne, degreaser
Uncertainties exist as to the potential effects on health when used in foods	Cottonseed oil, peanut oil, soy bean oil	

Names	Function	Code
Ozone (toxic form of oxygen)	Anti-microbial agent	☹
PABA (4-aminobenzoic acid)	Nutrient additive UV absorber	😐?
Pancreatin (from hog pancreas; of ANIMAL origin)	Food enzyme	😐?
Papain (enzyme from papaya, may be GE)	Food enzyme Meat tenderizer	😐?
Paprika (extracted from peppers)	Coloring (orange to red)	😊😊
para-Aminobenzoic acid (4-aminobenzoic acid)	Nutrient additive UV absorber	😐?
Paraffin wax (petroleum, coal, wood or shale oil derivative)	Coating Emollient	😐?
Paraldehyde (from the action of sulfuric acid on acetaldehyde)	Processing aid	☹

Potential Effects	Possible Food Use	Other Uses
Respiratory, cardiovascular, gastrointestinal, liver, skin, immuno and neurotoxicity; asthma; lung damage	Bottled water	
See 4-aminobenzoic acid	See 4-aminobenzoic acid	See 4-amino-benzoic acid
May cause allergic reactions in those allergic to pork	Liquid & dried egg whites, hydrolyzed animal, milk and vegetable proteins, instant cereals	Processing cosmetics, face peels
Considered to have health benefits; may cause allergic reactions; caused birth defects in animal studies	Instant cereals, sausage casings, bakery goods, dietary supplements	Skin creams, masks & scrubs
Believed safe in food use; may have beneficial health effects	Cheese slices, chicken pot pies, condiments, soup	Poultry feed
See 4-aminobenzoic acid	See 4-aminobenzoic acid	See 4-amino-benzoic acid
Believed nontoxic when pure; impurities can cause skin irritation and eczema	Chewing gum base, cheese, fresh fruits & vegetables	Lipstick, cold cream, mascara, protective cream
Neurotoxicity; hypnotic, sedative; can be habit forming	Candy, beverages, fats and oils, processing food additives, baked goods, instant coffee	

Names	Function	Code	
Pectin (from apple residue and citrus rind; on the NIH HSDB)	Stabilizer Thickener Emulsifier	☺	
Peppermint oil (from the plant *Mentha piperita*)	Flavoring	☺?	
Pepsin (digestive enzyme; from glandular layer of hog stomach; of ANIMAL origin)	Food enzyme	☺☺	
Petrolatum (petroleum jelly; from petroleum; on the NIH HSDB)	Release agent Polishing agent	☹	
Phenol (carbolic acid; from coal tar or petroleum; on the Canadian Hotlist; on the NIH HSDB)	Preservative	☹☹	
Phenylalanine (essential amino acid)	Nutrient additive	☺	

Potential Effects	Possible Food Use	Other Uses
Can lead to electrolyte and fluid loss in young children & the elderly with diarrhea; may provoke symptoms in those who react to MSG	Ice cream, fruit jellies & preserves, sherbet, jams, candy, sour cream, frozen desserts	Toothpaste, cosmetics, anti-diarrheal medicines
Can cause allergic reactions; hay fever; skin rash; allergic contact dermatitis	Various processed foods and beverages	Toothpaste, shaving cream, cigarettes
Believed safe in food use	Cottage cheese, cream cheese, hydrolyzed animal, milk and vegetable proteins	
Can interfere with digestion and absorption of essential nutrients; may discolor the skin in topical applications; allergic skin reactions	Bakery products, fresh fruits and vegetables	Lipstick, baby creams and lotions, eye shadow, wax depilatories
Ingestion can cause coma, paralysis; cardiovascular, respiratory, liver, developmental, reproductive, skin, kidney, gastrointestinal and neurotoxicity; toxic to aquatic organisms	Used in the manufacture of many food additives	Mouthwash, disinfectant, shaving cream, hand lotion, medical preparations, household surface cleaner
Believed safe in food use at low levels; those with phenylketonuria (PKU) should avoid	Dietary supplements	Hair conditioner

Names	Function	Code	
Phosphoric acid (made from phosphate rock; on the NIH HSDB)	Buffer	😐?	
Phosphorus oxychloride	Starch modifying agent	🙁	
Piperonal (synthetic)	Flavoring	😐?	
Polyacrylamide (polymer of acrylamide monomers; on the NIH HSDB)	Thickener	🙁	
Polydextrose (similar to cellulose)	Humectant Stabilizer	🙂	
Polyethylene glycol	De-foaming agent	😐?	
Polyglycerol esters of fatty acids (made from edible fats, oils and fatty acids; may be of ANIMAL origin; may be GE)	Emulsifier	🙂🙂	
Polyoxyethylene (40) monostearate (stearic acid & ethylene oxide)	Emulsifier Antifoaming agent	😐?	

Potential Effects	Possible Food Use	Other Uses
Believed safe in food use at low levels; excess may lead to tooth erosion and calcium loss in bones	Cheese products, soft drinks, jellies, sweets	Hair color, hand cleaner, nail polish, shampoo
Kidney, respiratory, skin and neurotoxicity	Modifier for food starch	
Believed safe in food use at low levels; large amounts can cause CNS depression; skin irritation; skin rash	Processed foods like beverages, ice cream, candy, baked goods	Perfumes, lipstick, soaps
Highly toxic; respiratory and neurotoxicity; skin irritation; can be absorbed through the skin	Washing fruits and vegetables; processing sugarcane	Blemish remover, moisturizer, tanning creams, adhesives
Believed safe in food use at low levels; excess may have a laxative effect; NRC	Low calorie foods, ice cream, yogurt, instant pudding mix, candy	Skin care products
Believed safe in food use; kidney and skin toxicity; may be contaminated with the carcinogen 1,4 dioxane	Processing of beet sugar and yeast, soft drinks	Antiperspirant, hair products, baby products, lipstick, toothpaste
Believed safe in food use	Vegetable oils, calorie-reduced margarine, unstandardized foods	
Skin tumors in mice; may facilitate the penetration of cancer-causing additives	Processed foods; frozen desserts	Hand cream and lotion

113

Names	Function	Code
Polyoxyethylene (20) sorbitan monooleate (polysorbate 80)	Emulsifier Thickener Stabilizer	☹
Polyoxyethylene (20) sorbitan monostearate (polysorbate 60)	Emulsifier Thickener Stabilizer	☹
Polyoxyethylene (20) sorbitan tristearate (polysorbate 65)	Emulsifier Antifoaming agent	☹
Polyoxyethylene (8) stearate (stearic acid & ethylene oxide; banned in some countries)	Emulsifier Thickener Stabilizer	☹
Polysorbate 60 (sorbitol and stearic acid chemically combined then sterilized with ethylene oxide)	Emulsifier Thickener Stabilizer	☹
Polysorbate 65	Emulsifier Antifoaming agent	☹
Polysorbate 80 (from sorbitol and oleic or stearic acid sterilized with ethylene oxide; on the NIH HSDB)	Emulsifier Thickener Stabilizer	☹
Polyvinyl polypyrrolidone (synthetic protein)	Clarifying agent	☹

Potential Effects	Possible Food Use	Other Uses
See polysorbate 80	See polysorbate 80	
See polysorbate 60	See polysorbate 60	
See polysorbate 65	See polysorbate 65	
Caused tumors and bladder stones in animal studies	Unstandardized bakery products	
Connected with the contaminants 1,4 dioxane and ethylene oxide known to cause cancer in animals	Cakes, cake mixes, icing, candy, beverage mixes, salad dressings	
Polysorbates can contain residues of harmful chemicals; can increase the absorption of fat soluble substances	Ice cream, cakes, frozen custard, cake icings and fillings, flavored milk, breath freshener products	
Connected with the contaminants 1,4 dioxane and ethylene oxide known to cause cancer in animals	Icing, frozen custard, sherbet, mayonnaise, ice cream, pickles, salad dressings	Suntan lotion, baby lotion, skin toner, toothpaste, filler in vaccines
See polyvinylpyrrolidone	Used to clarify sparkling wine and vinegar	Hairspray

Names	Function	Code	
Polyvinylpyrrolidone (PVP; povidone; synthetic; from petroleum by-products; on the NIH HSDB)	Stabilizer Clarifying agent	☹	
Ponceau 4R (cochineal Red A; azo dye; banned in some countries)	Coloring (red)	☹	
Ponceau SX (FD&C Red No. 4; azo dye; banned in foods in some countries)	Coloring	☹	
Potassium acetate (potassium salt of acetic acid)	Buffer Preservative	☺	
Potassium acid tartrate (potassium salt of tartaric acid)	Buffer	☺☺	
Potassium alginate (potassium salt of alginic acid)	Thickener Stabilizer	☺	
Potassium aluminum sulfate (aluminum potassium sulfate)	Firming agent Clarifying agent	😐?	
Potassium benzoate (synthetic; potassium salt of benzoic acid)	Preservative	😐?	

Potential Effects	Possible Food Use	Other Uses
Lung and kidney damage; gas; skin sensitization; gastrointestinal and liver toxicity; contact may cause allergic contact dermatitis; animal carcinogen	Fruit juice, beer, wine and vinegar manufacture	Hairspray, shave gel, shampoo, detergents, sunscreen, pharmaceuticals
Asthma; hay fever; hives; caution advised if aspirin sensitive; hyperactivity; suspected carcinogen	Jelly crystals, jam, cake mix, dessert toppings, tomato soup	
Caused adverse health effects in animal studies; not adequately tested for human consumption	Maraschino cherries, fruit peel, glace cherries	Cosmetics, hair rinse, perfume, mouthwash
People with impaired kidney function or cardiac disease may wish to avoid	Pickles, chutney, cheese, brown sauce, fruit sauce	Diuretics
See potassium tartrate	See potassium tartrate	
See alginates	Ice cream, yogurt, custard mix	
See aluminum potassium sulfate	See aluminum potassium sulfate	See aluminum potassium sulfate
Asthma; hives; eczema; allergic reactions; gastric irritation; caution advised if aspirin sensitive	Low-calorie jams and spreads, chili paste, glace cherries	Cosmetics

Names	Function	Code	
Potassium bicarbonate (carbonic acid)	Buffer Stabilizer	☺	
Potassium bisulfite	Preservative	☹	
Potassium bromate (on the Canadian Hotlist)	Maturing agent	☹	
Potassium carbonate (potash; from potassium hydroxide and carbon dioxide; on the NIH HSDB)	Buffer Leavening agent	☺?	
Potassium carrageenan	Thickener Stabilizer Emulsifier	☺?	
Potassium caseinate (potassium complexed with milk proteins (casein))	Texturizer	☺?	
Potassium chloride (extracted from sylvite or lake salt brines; on the NIH HSDB)	Yeast food Gelling agent	☺?	
Potassium citrate (potassium salt of citric acid)	Buffer Stabilizer	☺	

Potential Effects	Possible Food Use	Other Uses
Believed safe in food use; those with kidney or heart problems may wish to avoid	Confections, cocoa products, infant formula, margarine, processed cheese, baking powder	Shampoo, perm lotion, washing powder
See sulfites	Beer, wine, beverages, ketchup, pickles, relishes, fruit-pie mix	
Toxic by ingestion; adverse effects in animal studies including cancer; bleeding and inflammation of gums; mutagenic	Bread, white flour	Toothpaste, mouthwash
Believed safe in food use; irritation of skin & mucous membranes of eyes and upper respiratory tract	Cocoa products, baked goods, confections, processed cheese, cream cheese spread	Shampoo, soap, perm lotion
See carrageenan	See carrageenan	
Casein can cause allergic reactions and aggravate the symptoms of autism	Frozen custard, ice milk, ice cream, fruit sherbet	
Believed safe in food use at low levels; intestinal ulcers; cardiovascular, liver and respiratory toxicity; NRC	Unstandardized bakery foods, beer, ale, low sodium dietary foods	Cosmetics, household detergent
See citrates	Candy, jellies, preserves	

Names	Function	Code
Potassium fumarate (potassium bound to fumaric acid)	Acidifier	☺☺
Potassium furcelleran	Emulsifier Thickener	☺
Potassium gluconate (potassium salt of gluconic acid)	Sequestrant Buffer	☺
Potassium glutamate (may be GE)	Flavor enhancer	☹
Potassium hydroxide (lye; prepared from potassium chloride; on the NIH HSDB)	Emulsifier	☺?
Potassium iodate (potassium bound to iodine)	Dough conditioner Anti-caking agent	☺
Potassium iodide (potassium bound to iodine; on the NIH HSDB)	Dough conditioner Anti-caking agent	☺
Potassium lactate (potassium salt of lactic acid; may be of ANIMAL origin; may be GE)	Buffer Humectant	☺
Potassium metabisulfite (see sulfites)	Preservative Antioxidant	☹

Potential Effects	Possible Food Use	Other Uses
See fumaric acid	See fumaric acid	
See furcelleran	See furcelleran	
Believed safe in food use; mildly toxic by ingestion	Seltzer	
See monosodium glutamate	See monosodium glutamate	
Believed safe in food use; very corrosive; skin toxicity; tumors in mice when applied to the skin	Extracting color from annatto seed, cacao products	Hand lotion, cuticle removers (skin irritation and nail damage)
Believed safe in food use; caution advised if renal or thyroid function is impaired	Bread, bakery products	Animal feeds
Believed safe in food use; allergic reactions; caution advised if renal or thyroid function is impaired	Bread, bakery products, iodized table salt	Dye remover
Believed safe in food use; caution advised in those with lactose intolerance	Cookies, crackers, candy, foods for infants, cheese	Skin lotion, manicure lotion
Asthma; hives; behavioral problems; gastric irritation; anaphylaxis	Cheese and cheese products, home wine making kits	Bleaching straw, pet foods

Names	Function	Code
Potassium nitrate (saltpeter; from potassium chloride or hydroxide or carbonate and nitric acid; banned in foods in some countries; on the NIH HSDB)	Preservative Color fixative	☹
Potassium nitrite (banned in foods in some countries; see also nitrites in section 2)	Preservative Color fixative	☹
Potassium permanganate (synthetic)	Starch modifying agent	☹
Potassium phosphate (from phosphoric acid and potassium carbonate; on the NIH HSDB)	Buffer Stabilizer Sequestrant	☺
Potassium pyrophosphate (synthetic)	Sequestrant	☺
Potassium sorbate (from sorbic acid and potassium hydroxide; on the NIH HSDB)	Antioxidant Preservative	☺?
Potassium stearate (potassium salt of stearic acid; may be of ANIMAL origin)	De-foaming agent Emulsifier	☺☺

Potential Effects	Possible Food Use	Other Uses
May interfere with vitamin A absorption; may combine with amino acids in the stomach to form cancer-causing nitrosamines; NRC	Cured meats, dry sausage, ripened cheese, should not be added to baby foods	Toothpaste for sensitive teeth, processed animal foods, tobacco, matches
May combine with amino acids in the stomach to form cancer-causing nitrosamines; may cause stomach cancer; NRC	Bacon, preserved poultry products	Processed animal foods
Gastrointestinal, liver, respiratory and neurotoxicity	Modifier for food starch	Disinfectant
Believed safe in food use at low levels; caution advised if renal function is impaired	Frozen egg products, baking powder, yeast foods	Shampoo, facial cleanser, filler in vaccines, medicines
Believed safe in food use at low levels; excess may cause kidney damage, decrease in bone density	Meat tenderizers, prepared meats	Soaps, detergents
Allergic reactions; asthma; eye and skin irritation; behavioral problems	Bread, cheese, baked goods, cheesecake, wine making, chocolate	Moisturizer, washcloths, shampoo, cigarettes
Believed safe in food use	Chewing gum base; used in the brewing industry	Hand cream, hair conditioner, face wash, soaps

Names	Function	Code
Potassium sulfate (may be from potassium chloride and sulfuric acid or sulfur dioxide; on the NIH HSDB)	Buffer	☺
Potassium sulfite	Preservative Antioxidant	☹
Potassium tartrate (potassium salt of tartaric acid)	Buffer	☺?
Propane (n-propane; from petroleum or natural gas; on the NIH HSDB)	Propellant Aerator	☺?
Propionic acid (synthetic; may be from wood pulp & waste liquor or ethylene & CO; on the NIH HSDB)	Preservative	☺?
Propylene glycol (1,2-propanediol; synthetic, from propylene oxide; on the NIH HSDB)	Carrier or extraction solvent Humectant	☹
Propylene glycol alginate (synthetic; propylene glycol ester of alginic acid)	De-foaming agent Stabilizer Filler	☺?

Potential Effects	Possible Food Use	Other Uses
Believed safe in food use at low levels; ingesting large doses can cause severe gastrointestinal bleeding	Low sodium salt substitute, brewing industry	Deodorant soap, medicines, fertilizer
See sulfites	See sodium sulfite	
Should be avoided by people with impaired kidney or liver function, high blood pressure, edema or cardiac failure	Candy products, baking powder, honey wine	
May be narcotic in high concentrations; neurotoxicity; being reassessed for safety	Foamed and sprayed foods	Shaving cream, mousse, aerosol deodorants and antiperspirants
Migraines; skin irritation; headaches; toxic to aquatic organisms	Ice cream, bread, baked goods, sweets, processed cheeses	Perfume, lipstick, food wrappers
Skin and eye irritation; dry skin; respiratory, immuno, skin and neurotoxicity; CNS depression and kidney damage in animals	Candy, baked goods, chocolate products, sweetened coconut, toppings, food colors and flavors	Pet foods, suntan lotion, toothpaste, lipstick, baby lotion, cigarettes, antifreeze
Allergic reactions; avoid in pregnancy; see propylene glycol and alginates	Salad dressing, ice cream, frozen custard	Cosmetics

Names	Function	Code
Propylene glycol ether of methylcellulose	Thickener Emulsifier	☺?
Propylene glycol mono-esters & diesters of fats & fatty acids (may be GE)	Emulsifier Carrier or extraction solvent	☺?
Propyl gallate (synthetic; from n-propyl alcohol and 3,4,5-trihydroxybenzoic acid; may be used with BHA and BHT; on the NIH HSDB)	Antioxidant Preservative	☺?
Propylparaben (propyl-p-hydroxy benzoate; see parabens in section 2)	Preservative	☹
Propylene oxide (may be from potassium hydroxide and propylene chlorohydrin; on the NIH HSDB)	Starch modifying agent	☹☹
Propyl p-hydroxybenzoate (propylparaben; from propyl alcohol & p-hydroxybenzoic acid; on the NIH HSDB)	Preservative	☹
Protease (enzyme from bacteria or fungi; probably GE)	Food enzyme	☺

Potential Effects	Possible Food Use	Other Uses
See propylene glycol and methylcellulose	Candy, infant formula, icing, topping, ice cream, pickles, soup, dried mixed fruit	Contact dermatitis; Lactic acidosis;
See propylene glycol and mono- and diglycerides	Annatto butter color, oil-soluble annatto, annatto margarine color	
Allergic reactions; asthma; contact dermatitis; caution advised if aspirin sensitive	Mayonnaise, fats and oils, margarine, chewing gum, instant potato products	Cosmetic creams and lotions, tapes and labels in contact with food
See propyl-p-hydroxy benzoate	See propyl-p-hydroxy benzoate	See propyl-p-hydroxy benzoate
Gastrointestinal, immuno, liver, skin, developmental, reproductive and neurotoxicity; probable human carcinogen	Modifier for food starch	Shoe polish, waterproofing compounds, brake fluid, pesticide
Asthma; allergic reactions; skin redness, itching and swelling; hives; anaphylaxis	Beverages, baked goods, sweets, jellies, preserves, fruit flavoring	Baby products, mascara, makeup, shampoo
Believed safe in food use	Processed cheese, hydrolyzed animal, milk and vegetable protein, sausage casing, dough	

Names	Function	Code
Pyridoxine hydrochloride (form of vitamin B6; synthetic)	Nutrient additive	☺
Quillaia extract (quillaja extract; banned in foods in some countries)	Flavoring Foaming agent	☺
Quinine (quinoline alkaloid from cinchona bark)	Flavoring Local anesthetic	☺?
Quinoline (from aniline, acetaldehyde and formaldehyde)	Solvent	☹
Rapeseed oil (oil extracted from the seeds of a turnip-like herb; most likely GE, unless declared otherwise)	Emulsifier Stabilizer	☹
Rennet (rennin; enzyme from the stomach lining of calves; of ANIMAL origin; see chymosin)	Food enzyme Digestant	☺

Potential Effects	Possible Food Use	Other Uses
Believed safe in food use at low levels; those on L-dopa for Parkinson's Disease should use with caution	Infant foods, dietary supplements	Shampoo, hair conditioner, medications
Believed safe in food use at low levels; can cause gastrointestinal irritation; large doses can cause liver damage, respiratory failure, convulsions and coma	Soft drinks, ice cream, sweets, beverage mixes	Shampoo
Headache; tinnitus; skin rash; cardiovascular, liver and gastrointestinal toxicity	Beverages, tonic water	Hair products, cold remedies, sunscreens
Psoriasis; dermatitis; liver, gastrointestinal, respiratory & neurotoxicity; recognized carcinogen; hazardous to the environment, especially fish	Manufacture of synthetic food colors	Manufacture of cosmetic dyes, preservative for anatomical specimens
Acne-like skin eruptions; adverse health effects in animal studies including kidney and liver damage	Salad oils, cake mixes, peanut oil	
Believed safe in food use	Junket, cheese making	

Names	Function	Code	
Riboflavin (vitamin B2; may be GE)	Coloring (yellow or orange)	☺	
Rose hips extract (from the fruit of wild roses)	Flavoring	☺☺	
Roselle (extract from a herb native to South East Asia)	Flavoring Coloring (red)	☺☺	
Rosemary extract (from an evergreen shrub)	Flavoring Fragrance	☺	
Saccharin (hermesetas; may be prepared from toluenesulfonic acids, chlorine and ammonia; banned or restricted in foods in many countries; on the NIH HSDB)	Sweetener	☹	
Saffron (from the crocus plant, *Crocus sativus*)	Coloring (yellow to orange/brown)	☺☺	
Salicylates (salts of salicylic acid, benzyl, amyl, methyl, phenyl; found in fruits and vegetables)	Flavoring	☺?	

Potential Effects	Possible Food Use	Other Uses
Believed safe in food use; has beneficial effects in the body	Baby cereals, enriched breads, peanut butter, breakfast cereals	Multi-vitamin supplements
Rich in vitamin C	Natural flavoring used in organic foods	Skin cream, sun care products
Believed safe in food use	Jellies, tarts, apple jelly, non-carbonated beverages, fruit punch	
Considered to have beneficial health effects; may cause photosensitivity	Natural flavoring used in organic foods	Bubble bath, skin cream, shampoo
Diarrhea; diuresis; eczema; nausea; hives; headache; NRC; developmental and reproductive toxicity; suspected mutagen and carcinogen	Beverages, candy, table sweeteners, chewing gum, jams and jellies, dietetic foods	Chewable aspirin, toothpaste, pharmaceutical preparations
Believed safe in food use at low levels; has beneficial health effects	Jellies, icing sugar, caviar, jams, tomato sauce, pickles	Cosmetics, perfume, marking ink
Allergic reactions in people sensitive to aspirin; asthma; photoallergy; hyperactivity; kidney, cardiovascular and neurotoxicity; skin rash	Processed foods like ice cream, jam, cake mixes, chewing gum	Antiseptics, sunburn cream

Names	Function	Code
Salicylic acid (synthetic; may be derived by heating sodium phenate with carbon dioxide; one of the beta hydroxy acids; on the Canadian Hotlist; on the NIH HSDB)	Preservative Antiseptic	☹
Saponin (may be natural or synthetic)	Foaming agent	☺☺
Sassafras oil (volatile oil from sassafras plant; 80% safrole)	Flavoring Fragrance	😐?
Shellac (from resin produced by the lac insect)	Glazing agent	☺
Silica aerogel	Antifoaming agent	☺☺
Silicon dioxide (silica; component of rocks and sand)	Anti-caking agent	☺☺
Silver metal (a naturally occurring metal; on the Canadian Hotlist)	Coloring (metallic)	😐?
Smoke flavoring (prepared from smoke condensate)	Flavoring Antioxidant	😐?

Potential Effects	Possible Food Use	Other Uses
Large amounts absorbed can cause abdominal pain, vomiting, acidosis and skin rash; allergic reactions; dermatitis; suspected teratogen; aspirin-sensitive people should avoid	Various processed foods	Face cream, skin lotion, makeup, deodorant, suntan lotion, shampoo, making aspirin
Believed safe in food use	Beverage bases and mixes, soft drinks	Detergents
Dermatitis in sensitive people; unsafe in foods unless safrole-free; see safrole	Processed foods like beverages, ice cream, candy, baked goods	Perfume, soap, dentifrices, topical antiseptic
Believed safe in food use; allergic contact dermatitis; skin irritation	Candy, waxed fruit	Cosmetics, hair products, mascara, jewelry, tablets
Believed safe in food use	Beverages	Glass making
Believed safe in food use; silicon has beneficial health effects	Vegetable-oil-based cookware coating emulsions, dried egg products	Paper and paperboard products
Toxic in very large doses; should not be consumed; accumulates in tissues; argyria; kidney damage	External decoration on cakes, silver-colored almonds	Cosmetics, nail polish, soldering
Uncertainties exist regarding effects on human health; needs further studies	Cheese, soups, meats, crackers, seasonings	

Names	Function	Code
Sodium acetate (sodium salt of acetic acid)	Buffer Preservative	☺
Sodium acid phosphate (synthetic)	Sequestrant	☺
Sodium acid pyrophosphate (synthetic)	Leavening Sequestrant	☺
Sodium acid tartrate (synthetic)	Buffer	☺☺
Sodium alginate (sodium salt of alginic acid)	Thickener Stabilizer	☺
Sodium aluminosilicate (on the NIH HSDB)	Anti-caking agent	☺?
Sodium aluminum phosphate (synthetic)	Emulsifier Buffer	☺?
Sodium aluminum silicate (synthetic)	Anti-caking agent	☺?
Sodium aluminum sulfate (synthetic)	Bleaching agent	☺?

Potential Effects	Possible Food Use	Other Uses
Believed safe in food use; skin and eye irritation; moderate toxicity by ingestion	Sweets, jams, jellies, soup mixes, snack foods, cereals	Cosmetics, textiles, photographic and dye processes
Believed safe in food use at low levels; excess phosphorus can lead to heart, bone and kidney problems	Frozen desserts, cheeses	
Believed safe in food use at low levels; excess phosphorus can lead to heart, bone and kidney problems	Baking powder, canned seafood, frozen fish fillets, frozen crustacea, cream cheese spread	
Believed safe in food use	Baking powder	
See alginates	Frozen desserts, jams, fruit jelly preserves	Baby lotion, perms
Believed safe in food use at low levels; skin, eye and mucous membrane irritation; see aluminum	Beverage whitener, baking powder, dry soup mix	Dental compounds, dentifrices
Believed safe in food use at low levels; people with kidney or heart disease may wish to avoid or limit intake; see aluminum	Self-raising flour, various cheeses	
See sodium aluminosilicate	See sodium aluminosilicate	See sodium aluminosilicate
Believed safe in food use at low levels; see aluminum	Cereal flours	

Names	Function	Code
Sodium ascorbate (synthetic; sodium salt of ascorbic acid)	Antioxidant	☺☺
Sodium benzoate (from benzoic acid and sodium hydroxide; on the NIH HSDB)	Preservative	☹
Sodium bicarbonate (baking soda; synthetic, from water, sodium carbonate and carbon dioxide; on the NIH HSDB)	Leavening agent Neutralizer	😐?
Sodium bisulfite (synthetic)	Preservative Antioxidant	☹
Sodium calcium aluminosilicate (synthetic)	Anti-caking agent	😐?
Sodium carbonate (mostly synthetic, from sodium chloride and calcium carbonate using ammonia; on the NIH HSDB)	Buffer Anti-caking agent	😐?

Potential Effects	Possible Food Use	Other Uses
Believed safe in food use	Foods for infants, frozen fish, wine, vinegar, beer	Cosmetics
Asthma; hives; hay fever; contact dermatitis; mouth & skin irritation; hyperactivity; cardiovascular, liver, skin, gastrointestinal, kidney and neurotoxicity	Soft drinks, fruit juice, jam, condiments, baked goods, tomato paste, pickles, margarine	Toothpaste, body wash, shampoo, mouthwash, deodorant, diagnostic aid for liver function
Believed safe in foods at low levels; respiratory, kidney, gastrointestinal and liver toxicity; contact can cause forehead, scalp and hand rash	Pancake and biscuit mix, tomato soup, ice cream, sherbet, beverages, candies	Toothpaste, baby powder, hair color, shampoo, vaginal douches, laundry detergent
See sulfites; suspected mutagen	Gelatin, fruits, wines, manufacture of sulfite food preservatives	
See aluminum	Salt, dry mixes	
Believed safe in food use at low levels; large doses can cause gastro-intestinal bleeding, vomiting, diarrhea, shock and death; contact can cause scalp, forehead and hand rash; respiratory distress	Candies, flour products, ice cream mix, soup, jams, chocolate, malted milk powder	Toothpaste, mouthwash, soap, bath salts, vaginal douches, shampoo, paper manufacture, laundry detergent

Names	Function	Code	
Sodium carboxymethyl cellulose (made from cotton by-products; may be GE)	Thickener Stabilizer	☺?	
Sodium carrageenan	Thickener Stabilizer Emulsifier	☹?	
Sodium caseinate (sodium complexed with milk proteins [casein])	Texturizer	☺?	
Sodium cellulose glycolate	Thickener Stabilizer	☹?	
Sodium chloride (table salt; may contain aluminum as an anti-caking agent; on the NIH HSDB)	Preservative Flavor enhancer	☹?	
Sodium chlorite (synthetic)	Starch modifying agent	☹	
Sodium citrate (from sodium sulfate and calcium citrate; on the NIH HSDB)	Buffer Emulsifier	☺	
Sodium diacetate (synthetic)	Preservative	☺	

Potential Effects	Possible Food Use	Other Uses
Poorly absorbed; flatulence; large amounts can cause diarrhea and abdominal cramps; caused cancer and tumors in animal studies	Pickles, salad dressing, ice cream, cottage cheese	Hair lotions, hand cream, laxatives, toothpaste, tobacco
See carrageenan	See carrageenan	
Casein can cause allergic reactions and aggravate the symptoms of autism	Ice cream, ice milk, fruit sherbet, soups, stews	
See sodium carboxymethyl cellulose	See sodium carboxymethyl cellulose	
Believed safe in small amounts; excess may lead to high blood pressure, increased risk of stroke; cardiovascular toxicity	Added to a wide range of processed foods during manufacture	Mouthwash, body wash, bubble bath, dentifrices, liquid hand soap, shampoo
Gastrointestinal, liver and developmental toxicity	Modifier for food starch	Agricultural chemicals, paper & textile industry
See citrates; may interfere with the urinary excretion of some drugs making them either less effective or more potent	Infant formula, cottage cheese, ice cream, evaporated milk, jams, preserves, fruit jellies	Shampoo, hair conditioner, laundry stain remover
See sodium acetate	Bread, baked goods	

Names	Function	Code	
Sodium erythorbate (synthetic)	Antioxidant	☺☺	
Sodium ferrocyanide (synthetic; from the reaction of cyanide with iron sulfate)	Anti-caking agent	☺☺	
Sodium fumarate (synthetic)	Buffer Antioxidant	☺☺	
Sodium furcelleran	Emulsifier Thickener Stabilizer	☺	
Sodium gluconate (sodium salt of gluconic acid)	Buffer Sequestrant	☺	
Sodium hexametaphosphate (synthetic)	Emulsifier Sequestrant	☺?	
Sodium hydroxide (caustic soda; made by electrolysis of sodium chloride brine; on the NIH HSDB)	Emulsifier	☺	
Sodium hypochlorite (from sodium hydroxide and chlorine; on the NIH HSDB)	Preservative Bleaching agent	☹	

Potential Effects	Possible Food Use	Other Uses
Believed safe in food use	See sodium ascorbate	See sodium ascorbate
Believed safe in food use	Salts and condiments, processing wine	
See fumaric acid	See fumaric acid	
See furcelleran	See furcelleran	See furcelleran
Believed safe in food use; people with heart disease or high blood pressure may wish to avoid or limit consumption	Cream cheese spread, processed cheese	Metal cleaner, paint stripper, metal plating, rust remover
Believed safe in food use at low levels; neurotoxicity; excess phosphorus can lead to heart, bone and kidney problems	Ice cream, processed cheese, infant formula, breakfast cereals	Bubble bath, bath salts, shampoo
Believed safe in food use; contact can cause dermatitis; hazardous when concentrated	Modifier for food starch, glazing of pretzels, refining of vegetable oils	Shampoo, hand cleaner, body wash, toothpaste, drain cleaner
Ingestion can severely affect mucous membranes, esophagus and stomach; skin, cardiovascular and neurotoxicity	Washing of cottage cheese curd, modifier for food starch	Household bleach, pool and spa chemicals, drain cleaner, mildew remover

Names	Function	Code	
Sodium iso-ascorbate (erythorbic acid)	Antioxidant Preservative	☺	
Sodium lactate (sodium salt of lactic acid)	Humectant Bulking agent	☺	
Sodium lauryl sulfate (synthetic, by sulfation of lauryl alcohol and neutralization with sodium carbonate or sodium hydroxide; on the NIH HSDB)	Emulsifier Whipping agent Surfactant	☹	
Sodium metabisulfite (synthetic; from sodium bisulfite, or sodium carbonate and sulfur dioxide; on the NIH HSDB; see sulfites)	Preservative	☹	
Sodium nitrate (from sodium carbonate and nitric acid; banned in foods in some countries; on the NIH HSDB)	Preservative	☹	
Sodium nitrite (synthetic; banned in foods in some countries; on the NIH HSDB; see nitrites in section 2)	Preservative	☹	

Potential Effects	Possible Food Use	Other Uses
See erythorbic acid	See erythorbic acid	See erythorbic acid
Believed safe in food use; people with lactose intolerance may wish to avoid	Cookies, crackers, uncured hams, margarine	Moisturizer, skin toner, face wash, diaper rash cream
Moderately toxic; mucous membrane, eye and skin irritation; eczema; dry skin; mouth ulcers; liver and gastrointestinal toxicity; toxic to aquatic organisms	Dried, liquid and frozen egg whites, cake mixes, marshmallows	Bubble bath, toothpaste, hair conditioner, liquid hand and body wash, body soap, shampoo
Asthma (life threatening attacks); hay fever; chronic hives; atopic dermatitis; anaphylaxis; toxic to aquatic organisms	Bread and flour products, jellies, dried fruits, tomato paste, maraschino cherries, salad ingredients	Hair color, pet foods, deodorant, stain remover, pharmaceuticals
Dizziness; headaches; vomiting; migraine; nausea; cardiovascular and respiratory toxicity, NRC	Manufactured meats, dry sausage, ripened cheese, prosciutto ham	Processed animal foods, fertilizers, explosives
Headaches; dizziness; nausea; gastrointestinal, cardiovascular, kidney, developmental, respiratory and neurotoxicity; NRC; toxic to aquatic organisms	Canned, cured, manufactured and pressed meats, sausages, bacon	Anticorrosive in some cosmetics, floor polish, oven cleaner, pet foods

Names	Function	Code
Sodium phosphate (sodium salt of phosphoric acid)	Buffer Sequestrant	☺
Sodium potassium copper chlorophyllin	Characterization	☺☺
Sodium potassium tartrate (sodium and potassium salt of tartaric acid; Rochelle salt)	Buffer Stabilizer	☺
Sodium pyrophosphate (synthetic)	Sequestrant Emulsifier	☺
Sodium salt of methyl-p-hydroxy benzoic acid (sodium salt of methylparaben; see parabens in section 2)	Preservative	☹
Sodium silicate water glass; silicic acid bound to sodium; on the NIH HSDB)	Anti-caking agent Corrosion inhibitor	😐?
Sodium sorbate (sodium salt of sorbic acid)	Preservative	😐?

Potential Effects	Possible Food Use	Other Uses
Believed safe in foods at low levels; contact can cause skin irritation; erythema; blisters	Frozen desserts, noodle and macaroni products, cheese spread, sherbet	Toothpaste, shampoo, dish washing liquid
Believed safe in food use	Breath freshener products in candy, tablet or gum form	
Believed safe in food use; people with edema, high blood pressure, cardiac failure, kidney or liver damage advised to avoid	Candies, jams, fruit jelly preserves, cheese, manufacture of baking powder	Silvering of mirrors, mouthwash, cathartic in medicinal use
See sodium acid pyrophosphate	Bacon, canned ham, processed cheese, sherbet	
See methylparaben	See methylparaben	See methylparaben
Ingestion causes vomiting and diarrhea; skin and mucous membrane irritation	Preserved eggs, bottled water	Depilatories, protective skin creams
Allergic reactions; kidney, liver and blood pressure problems; fluid retention	Frozen pizza, pie fillings, cheese, cheesecake, cheese spread, chocolate syrup	Food packaging

Names	Function	Code
Sodium stearate (over 90% stearic acid; from sodium hydroxide and stearic acid; on the NIH HSDB)	Emulsifier Gelling agent Plasticizer	☺?
Sodium stearoyl lactylate (sodium stearoyl-2-lactylate; from lactic acid and fatty acids; may be of ANIMAL origin; may be GE)	Emulsifier Stabilizer	☺☺
Sodium stearyl fumarate (may be from corn, milk, soy or peanuts; probably GE)	Dough conditioner	☺
Sodium sulfate (sodium salt of sulfuric acid; on the NIH HSDB)	Buffer Preservative	☺?
Sodium sulfite (synthetic; sodium salts of sulfurous acid; on the NIH HSDB; see sulfites)	Preservative Antioxidant Anti-browning agent	☹
Sodium tartrate (sodium salt of tartaric acid)	Buffer Preservative	☺☺
Sodium thiosulfate (synthetic)	Antioxidant Stabilizer	☺?

Potential Effects	Possible Food Use	Other Uses
Believed safe in food use at low levels; excess consumption (of stearic acid) may increase the risk of diabetes mellitus type 2	Chewing gum	Soap, toothpaste, deodorant sticks, suppositories, plastics
Believed safe in food use at low levels	Cookies, crackers, bread, cakes, cake icings, fillings and toppings	Moisturizer, anti-aging cream
Believed safe in food use	Bread, bakery products	
Believed safe in foods at low levels; skin irritation; gastrointestinal irritation; people with poor kidney or liver function should avoid	Chewing gum base, cookies, crackers, tuna fish, frozen mushrooms	Manufacture of dyes, soap, detergents, glass and paper
Asthma; gastric irritation; skin rash; nausea; diarrhea; destroys vitamin B content in food; those with impaired liver or kidney function should avoid	Cut fruits, dried fruit, maraschino cherries, prepared fruit pie mix, frozen apples, canned flaked tuna	Hair dye
Believed safe in food use	Cheese, artificially sweetened jelly, meat products	
See sodium sulfate	Frozen French fries, sliced potatoes, salt	Treatment for ringworm and mange in animals

Names	Function	Code	
Sodium tripolyphosphate (synthetic)	Texturizer Sequestrant	☺	
Sorbic acid (mostly synthetic from chemicals such as acetaldehyde and ketene; on the NIH HSDB)	Preservative Humectant	☺?	
Sorbitan monostearate (synthesized from sorbitol and stearic acid; may be of ANIMAL origin; may be GE)	Emulsifier Glazing agent	☺	
Sorbitan trioleate (from sorbitol and oleic acid; may be of ANIMAL origin)	Emulsifier	☺?	
Sorbitan tristearate (prepared from sorbitol and stearic acid; may be of ANIMAL origin; may be GE)	Emulsifier	☺	
Sorbitol, sorbitol syrup (may be synthesized from glucose from corn sugar; may be GE; on the NIH HSDB)	Humectant Sweetener	☺?	

Potential Effects	Possible Food Use	Other Uses
Believed safe in food use at low levels; excess may cause depletion of calcium; skin irritation	Frozen seafood	Soaps, bubble bath
Allergic reactions; asthma; contact dermatitis; hives, erythema; skin irritation; behavioral problems	Frozen pizza, pie fillings, cheese, cheesecake, cheese spread, chocolate syrup	Pet foods, makeup remover, toothpaste, mouthwash
Believed safe in food use at low levels; high levels in the diet can cause intralobular fibrosis, growth retardation, liver enlargement	Candy, ice cream, flavored milk, bakery wares, cake mix, icing	Cosmetic cream and lotion, suntan cream, skin cream, deodorant
See sorbitol; believed safe in cosmetic use	Sausage casings	Makeup, skin cream, blusher, concealer
Believed safe in food use at low levels; high levels in the diet can cause intralobular fibrosis, growth retardation, liver enlargement	Compounded chocolate, oil toppings, cake mixes	Insecticides, nail strengthening cream
Excess intake can cause intestinal cramps; diarrhea; bloating; gastrointestinal disturbance; cataracts; may alter absorption of drugs so they are either more toxic or less effective	Candies, dried fruit, chewing gum, chocolate, lollipops, sweetening agent for diabetics	Hair conditioner, hairspray, shave gel, shampoo, mouthwash, toothpaste, filler in vaccines, antifreeze

Names	Function	Code
Soybean oil (soyabean oil; may be GE)	Emollient	☺?
Spermaceti wax (from the head of the sperm whale)	Glazing and polishing agent	☺
Splenda (synthetic)	Artificial sweetener	☺?
Squalene (shark liver oil; of ANIMAL origin)	Nutrient additive Emollient	☺☺
Stannous chloride (chloride of the metal tin)	Antioxidant	☺
Starch, food, modified (synthetic; starch treated with chemicals, some of which are toxic; may be GE)	Thickener Binder	☹
Stearic acid (may be synthetic from cottonseed and other vegetable oils; may be of ANIMAL origin [tallow]; may be GE; on the NIH HSDB)	Release agent Plasticizer	☺?

Potential Effects	Possible Food Use	Other Uses
Excess consumption can cause goiter, flatulence, indigestion, and allergic reactions; pimples; hair damage in topical use	Soy sauce, margarine, soy products	Body soap, skin cream, lipstick, moisturizer, body wash
Believed safe in food use at low levels	Candies	Hair color, skin cleansing cream, hair conditioner
See sucralose	See sucralose	
Considered to have beneficial health effects	Dietary supplements	Skin care products, fixative in perfumes
Believed safe in food use at low levels; skin and mucous membrane irritation; toxic to aquatic organisms	Canned and bottled asparagus, canned soft drinks	Dye manufacture
Questions arise concerning adverse effects on the body of chemicals used to treat starch, especially in infants	Processed foods, baby foods	Cosmetics, cigarettes
Believed safe in food use at low levels; excess intake may increase the risk of diabetes mellitus type 2; sensitizer for those with allergies; bioaccumulates in aquatic organisms	Candies, chewing gum, baked goods	Mascara, makeup, skin cream, shaving cream, baby lotion, bar soap, moisturizer, food packaging

Names	Function	Code	
Stearyl citrate (ester of stearyl alcohol and citric acid; of ANIMAL origin)	Sequestrant	☺	
Stearyl monoglyceridyl citrate (synthetic)	Stabilizer	☺	
Sterculia gum (karaya gum)	Thickener Stabilizer	☺?	
Stevia; stevioside (extract from the leaves of a South American plant)	Sweetener	☺	
Succinic acid (synthetic; from acetic or malic acid)	Buffer Neutralizer Flavoring	☺	
Succinic anhydride (synthetic)	Starch modifying agent	☺☺	
Sucralose (synthetically prepared from sugar and chlorine)	Artificial sweetener	☺?	
Sucrose acetate isobutyrate (synthetic; from sucrose, acetic acid and isobutyric anhydrides; on the NIH HSDB)	Emulsifier Stabilizer	☺	

Potential Effects	Possible Food Use	Other Uses
See citrates	Margarine	
See citrates	Shortening	
See karaya gum	See karaya gum	See karaya gum
Believed safe in foods; believed to have benefits to health; in animal studies it proved toxic to pregnant rodents and had affect on the kidneys	Dietary supplement	Shampoo, hair rinse
Believed safe in food use; excess may have a laxative effect	Used in food processing	Perfumes, mouthwash, lacquers
Believed safe in food use	Modifier for food starch	
Adverse health effects such as enlarged liver & kidneys and thymus shrinkage have been reported in animal studies; doubts exist about the safety of this chemical	Candies, diet soft drinks, baked goods, desserts, chewing gum	
Believed safe in foods; produced non-permanent liver changes in dogs but not in other species	Citrus flavored beverages	Nail polish

Names	Function	Code
Sucrose esters of fatty acids (from sucrose and fatty acids; may be of ANIMAL origin; may be GE)	Emulsifier Stabilizer	☺
Sulfites (ammonium, potassium and sodium salts of sulfurous acid)	Preservative Antioxidant	☹
Sulfur dioxide (produced by burning sulfur)	Preservative	☹
Sulfuric acid (battery acid; may be from sulfur, pyrite, hydrogen sulfide, smelter gases or gypsum; on the NIH HSDB)	Buffer	☺
Sulfurous acid (solution of sulfur dioxide in water)	Buffer Preservative	☹
Sunset Yellow FCF (FD&C Yellow No. 6)	Coloring (orange/yellow)	☹

Potential Effects	Possible Food Use	Other Uses
Believed safe in foods at low levels; large doses can cause nausea, bloating, diarrhea, gas, abdominal pain; can facilitate uptake of food allergens	Margarine, dairy desserts, chewing gum, chocolate, mayonnaise	Moisturizer
Acute asthma; anaphylactic shock; diarrhea; nausea; death; kidney, respiratory, skin and immunotoxicity; may destroy vitamin B1	Dried fruit, gelatin, wines, condiments, soft drinks, dried or dehydrated coconut, jam, vinegar, potato products	Making cellophane for food packaging
Asthma; bronchospasm; bronchoconstriction; hypotension; anaphylaxis; bronchitis; cardiovascular, gastrointestinal, liver and neurotoxicity; destroys vitamins A and B1 in food; animal mutagen	Dried fruit, beer, cider, fruit juice, gelatin, wines, pickles, soft drinks, dried or dehydrated coconut, vinegar	Pulp and paper manufacture, textile bleaching agents, pet foods
Believed safe in food use; corrosive and hazardous when concentrated	Used to modify starch, brewing industry	Drain cleaner, lead-acid batteries
Gastrointestinal and liver toxicity; toxic by inhalation & ingestion; tissue irritation	Gelatin, fruits, wines, manufacture of sulfite food preservatives	Paper making
See FD&C Yellow No. 6	See FD&C Yellow No. 6	

Names	Function	Code	
Talc (talcum powder; magnesium silicate; from natural talc deposits)	Anti-caking agent	☹	
Tannic acid	Flavoring Clarifying agent	☺?	
Tartaric acid (by-product of the wine industry)	Antioxidant Sequestrant	☺	
Tartrazine (FD&C Yellow No. 5)	Coloring (lemon yellow to orange)	☹	
TBHQ (tertiary butyl hydroquinone)	Antioxidant	☹	
Tertiary butylhydroquinone (TBHQ; from quinone [from coal-tar] and butane [from petroleum]; banned in foods in some countries; on the Canadian Hotlist; on the NIH HSDB)	Antioxidant	☹	
Tetrasodium pyrophosphate (TSPP; from phosphoric acid and sodium carbonate; on the NIH HSDB)	Emulsifier Sequestrant	☺?	

Potential Effects	Possible Food Use	Other Uses
Cough; stomach problems; respiratory problems; suspected carcinogen (stomach & ovarian cancer)	Chocolate, chewing gum base, condiments, candy, polished rice	Eye makeup, bath powder, baby powder, animal feed
Believed safe in food use at low levels; suspected of being a weak carcinogen	Processed foods like beverages, ice cream, candy, baked goods	Sunscreen, eye lotion, antiperspirant
Believed safe in food use at low levels; laxative effect from excess	Candy, jam, fruit jelly, fruit drink, baking powder, fruit juice, dried egg whites	Denture powder, hair rinses, nail bleaches, depilatories
See FD&C Yellow No. 5	See FD&C Yellow No. 5	See FD&C Yellow No. 5
See tertiary butyl hydroquinone	See tertiary butyl hydroquinone	See tertiary butyl hydroquinone
Hydroquinone may cause skin, gastrointestinal, liver, reproductive, immuno, cardiovascular and neurotoxicity; birth defects; delirium; allergic contact dermatitis; suspected carcinogen and mutagen	Edible oils and oil emulsions, potato chips	Suntan lotion, hair coloring, antiperspirant, deodorant
Moderately toxic; ingestion can cause nausea, diarrhea and vomiting; skin and eye irritation	Ice cream, processed cheese	Toothpaste, hair color, laundry detergent, dyeing textiles

Names	Function	Code	
Thaumatin (extracted from the fruit of a West African plant)	Flavor enhancer Sweetener	☺☺	
THBP (2-3-4 trihydroxybutyrophenone)	Antioxidant	☹	
Theobroma oil (derived from cacao bean)	Emollient Botanical additive	☺	
Theobromine (alkaloid found in cacao beans closely related to caffeine)	Botanical additive	☺	
Thiamine hydrochloride (synthetic; form of vitamin B1; thiamine and hydrochloric acid)	Nutrient additive	☺☺	
Thiamine mononitrate (thiamine nitrate; form of vitamin B1; synthetic)	Nutrient additive	☺☺	
Thymol (obtained from essential oil of lavender and others)	Flavoring Additive Fragrance	☺?	
Titanium dioxide (may be obtained from ilmenite or rutile; may contain Nanoparticles, see glossary; on the NIH HSDB)	Coloring (white) Opacifier	☺?	
Tocopherol (vitamin E; may be from vegetable oils or wheat germ; may be synthetic; may be GE; on the NIH HSDB)	Antioxidant	☺	

Potential Effects	Possible Food Use	Other Uses
Believed safe in food use	Chewing gum, Japanese seasonings?	
See trihydroxybutyrophenone	See trihydroxy-butyrophenone	See trihydroxy-butyrophenone
Allergic reactions in sensitive people; acne	Candy	Soap, cosmetics, pharmaceuticals
Believed safe in food use at low levels; stimulates the CNS; toxic to dogs	Chocolate products	Skin conditioner in cosmetics, pharmaceuticals
Believed safe in food use; considered to have many health benefits	Breakfast cereals, baby cereals, enriched flours, dietary supplements	Hair conditioner
Believed safe in food use; considered to have many health benefits	Enriched flour, dietary supplements	
Dizziness, vomiting, and nausea from ingestion; allergic reactions; neurotoxicity	Processed foods like beverages, ice cream, candy, baked goods, chewing gum	Cosmetics, aftershave, mouthwash
Believed safe in food use; may cause skin irritation; reproductive toxicity; limited evidence of cancer in animal studies	Sugar-coated candy, sweets, chewing gum, icing sugar, jam, jellies	Bath powder, bar soap, lipstick, face powder, toothpaste, body wash, sunscreen, mascara
Believed safe in food use; freezing may destroy it; high daily doses may produce adverse symptoms	Dairy blend, margarine, salad oil, reduced fat spread, dietary supplements	Deodorant, baby oil, mascara, hand and body lotion, lipstick

Names	Function	Code	
Tragacanth gum (derived from the plant *Astragalus gummifer*)	Thickener Emulsifier	☺	
Triacetin (glyceryl triacetate)	Carrier or extraction solvent	☺	
Triethyl citrate (from citric acid and ethanol; on the NIH HSDB)	Whipping agent Plasticizer	☺	
Trihydroxybutyrophenone (2-3-4 trihydroxybutyrophenone, THBP; may not appear on food labels)	Antioxidant	☹	
Trypsin (digestive enzyme; from hog pancreas; of ANIMAL origin)	Food enzyme	☺☺	
Turmeric (tumeric; from an East Indian herb)	Coloring (orange/yellow) Flavoring	☺☺	
Urea (carbamide; synthetic, from ammonia, carbon monoxide and sulfur; on the Canadian Hotlist)	Browning agent Humectant	☺?	

Potential Effects	Possible Food Use	Other Uses
Believed safe in food use at low levels; adverse effects such as asthma, abdominal pain, contact dermatitis, dyspnea, anaphylaxis and constipation are rare	Sauces, fruit jelly, salad dressing, candies, icings	Shaving cream, blush, toothpaste, foundation
See glyceryl triacetate	See glyceryl triacetate	See glyceryl triacetate
See citrates	Liquid and frozen egg white; dried egg	Hairspray, perfume base
Not adequately tested for human health effects; the FDA has requested further studies	Oily and fatty foods or may migrate into foods from packaging	Manufacture of food packaging materials
Believed safe in food use	Hydrolyzed animal, milk and vegetable proteins, enzyme supplements	Drug treatment for indigestion
Believed safe in food use; reported to have many beneficial effects on health	Oleomargarine, sausage casings, pickles, soups, condiments, shortening	
Allergic reactions in some people; dermatitis; thinning of the epidermis; redness & irritation of skin and eyes	Pretzels, chewing gum, yeast-raised bakery products	Body wash, dishwashing liquid, shampoo

Names	Function	Code	
Vanillin (synthetic; from eugenol, guaiacol or wood pulp waste; may be GE; on the NIH HSDB)	Flavoring	😐?	
Vegetable carbon (usually from burnt vegetable matter but may be of ANIMAL origin; may be GE; banned in foods in some countries)	Coloring (black)	😐?	
Waxes (from petroleum, animals, plants and insects; can contain pesticides; may be of ANIMAL origin)	Film former Emollient	😐?	
Wintergreen oil (methyl salicylate)	Flavoring Disinfectant	☹	
Xanthan gum (may be GE)	Thickener Emulsifier	😊😊	
Xanthophyll (carotenoid from flower petals)	Coloring (yellow)	😊😊	
Xylitol (formally from Birch wood, now made from waste products from the pulp industry)	Sweetener Humectant Stabilizer	😊	

Potential Effects	Possible Food Use	Other Uses
Allergic reactions; eye, skin and mucous membrane irritation, skin pigmentation	Processed foods like beverages, ice cream, candy, baked goods, chocolate, margarine	Perfume, makeup remover, drugs, cigarettes, dentifrices
Mildly toxic by ingestion, skin contact and inhalation; may be carcinogenic	Concentrated fruit juice, jams, jelly beans, licorice, candy	Cosmetics
Believed safe in cosmetic use; may cause allergic reactions depending on source and purity	Coatings on fresh vegetables and fruit, food packaging materials	Cosmetics, hair-grooming preparations, lipstick
See methyl salicylate; toxic to aquatic organisms	See methyl salicylate	See methyl salicylate
Believed safe in food use	Jellies, sweets, dairy products, breakfast cereal, salad dressing	Toothpaste, eye cream, mascara, cigarettes
Believed safe in food use	Processed foods	Skin conditioner
Believed safe in food use at low levels; reported to have beneficial effects on health; large doses may cause diarrhea and flatulence; tumors in animal studies	Ice cream, chocolate, jams, candy, chewing gum, toffee, mints	Toothpaste

Names	Function	Code	
Zein (protein found in corn; by-product of corn processing; probably GE)	Coating agent	☺	
Zinc sulfate (synthetic; reaction between zinc and sulfuric acid; on the NIH HSDB)	Nutrient additive	☺?	

Potential Effects	Possible Food Use	Other Uses
Believed safe in food use	Coating for various foods	Face masks, nail polish, plastics, coatings, inks, adhesives
Respiratory, cardiovascular, gastrointestinal, liver and developmental toxicity; allergic reactions	Dietary supplements, migration into foods from paperboard containers	Eye lotion, skin tonic, aftershave, shaving cream, paint coloring

SECTION 2
COSMETIC INGREDIENTS

Names	Function	Code	
Acetarsol (acetarsone)	Anti-microbial	☺?	
Acetonitrile (methylacyanide; precursor of cyanide; on the Canadian Hotlist)	Solvent	☹☹	
Acid colors e.g. acid red 14 (black, blue, brown, green, orange, red, violet, yellow; synthetic coal tar/azo dyes)	Colorant	☹	
Acrylamide and acrylamide copolymer (acrylamide is derived from acrylonitrile and sulfuric acid)	Film former Thickener	☹	
Allantoin (can be extracted from uric acid; may be of ANIMAL origin)	Anti-microbial Oral care agent	☺☺	
Alpha hydroxy acids (AHA's; glycolic acid, lactic acid, tartaric acid, malic acid, citric acid, salicyclic acid, L-alpha hydroxy acid, mixed fruit acids and others; on the Canadian Hotlist)	Exfoliant	☹	

Potential Effects	Cosmetic Uses	Other Uses
Sensitization; allergic reactions; lethal dose in mice is only 0.004g/kg of body weight	Mouthwash, toothpaste, feminine hygiene products	
Nervous system poison; skin irritation; gastrointestinal and liver toxicity; suspected teratogen; fatal if swallowed	Artificial nails remover	Packaging materials, extraction processes
Many can cause skin, eye and mucous membrane irritation; see azo dyes and coal tar	Tints and dyes for hair coloring	
Toxic by skin absorption; acrylamide may cause liver, reproductive & neurotoxicity; carcinogenic; hazardous in the environment; especially harmful to fish	Nail polish, face masks, cosmetics	Manufacture of dyes & adhesives, permanent-press fabrics
May accelerate cell growth promoting healing of fractures, scars, wounds; may alleviate psoriasis	Cold cream, hand lotion, hair lotion, aftershave lotion, hair conditioner, lipstick, baby lotion	
Long term skin damage; swelling, especially around the eyes; skin discoloration; itchiness; photosensitivity; rashes; skin blistering; may increase risk of skin cancer	Skin peels (do not use on children or infants), skin toner, face and body cream, cuticle softener, skin cleanser, skin improvers, shampoo	

169

Names	Function	Code	
Aluminum acetate (mixture including acetic acid and boric acid)	Anti-microbial	☹	
Aluminum chlorohydrate (synthetic)	Deodorant agent	☹	
Ammonium laureth sulfate (synthetic)	Surfactant	☺?	
Ammonium lauryl sulfate (synthetic; from n-dodecyl alcohol, chlorosulfonic acid and ammonia; on the NIH HSDB)	Surfactant Foaming agent	☺?	
Ammonium sulfate (ammonium salt; on the NIH HSDB)	Surfactant Cleanser	☹	
Ammonium thioglycolate (ammonium salt of thioglycolic acid; on the Canadian Hotlist)	Antioxidant	☹	

Potential Effects	Cosmetic Uses	Other Uses
Severe sloughing of the skin; skin rash; ingestion of large doses can cause diarrhea, nausea, vomiting and bleeding; see also aluminum in section 1	Antiperspirant, deodorant, protective creams	Waterproofing, fabric finishes, dye for furs
Contact allergic reactions; hair follicle infections; irritation of abraded skin; see also aluminum in section 1	Antiperspirant, deodorant	Pharmaceuticals
May be contaminated with carcinogenic nitrosamines	Shampoo, bubble bath, hand wash, body wash	Dishwashing liquid, detergent
Repeated use may dry the skin; eye and skin irritation; may cause contamination with nitrosamines	Shampoo, bubble bath, liquid hand and body wash, toothpaste, bath gel	Dishwashing liquid, car wash detergent, rug shampoo
Dry & denatured hair; liver, respiratory & neurotoxicity; fatal to rats fed large doses	Hair perm lotion, body wash	Tanning, fertilizer, filler in vaccines
Severe burns and blistering of the skin; hair breakage; cumulative irritant; severe allergic reactions; lethal to mice in large injected doses	Hair straightener, depilatories, hair perm lotion	

Names	Function	Code
Amyl dimethyl PABA (Padimate A; synthetic)	UV absorber	☹
Aniline and aniline dyes (coal tar dyes; derived mostly from nitrobenzene or chlorobenzene; on the Canadian Hotlist; on the NIH HSDB)	Organic base	☹☹
Ascorbyl palmitate (derived form ascorbic acid)	Preservative Antioxidant	☺
Azo dyes (extract from coal tar or crude oil; see coal tar)	Colorant	☹☹
Balsam Peru (extract from South American tree)	Antiseptic	☺?
Basic colors e.g. basic red 51 (many are azo or coal tar dyes or made from hazardous chemicals; some are on the Canadian Hotlist)	Colorant	☹

Potential Effects	Cosmetic Uses	Other Uses
May cause sensitization; may increase breast cancer cell division; mutagenic in sunlight; estrogenic; endocrine disruption; suspected carcinogen	Sunscreen (should not be used on infants under 6 months of age), makeup, hair conditioner	
Cardiovascular, respiratory, gastrointestinal, liver, kidney and neurotoxicity; aniline is a recognized carcinogen	Hair dyes, perfumes	Manufacture of drugs, resins, paint remover, adhesives
Some palmitates may cause contact dermatitis	Cosmetic creams and lotions	
Skin contact can cause hives, asthma; hay fever; allergic reactions; suspected bladder cancer; may be absorbed through the skin	Non-permanent hair rinses and tints	Synthetic colorings foods and beverages
Skin irritation, stuffy nose; contact dermatitis; common sensitizer; may cross-react with benzoic acid and others	Cream hair rinse, face masks, perfume	Cigarettes
See aniline dyes, azo dyes, and coal tar	Hair dyes and tints, shampoo	Some are used for coloring paper and fabrics

Names	Function	Code	
Benzalkonium chloride (BAK; on the Canadian Hotlist; on the NIH HSDB)	Preservative Detergent	☹	
Beta hydroxy acids (BHA's; salicylic acid, beta hydroxy butanoic acid, tropic acid, trethocanic acid)	Exfoliant	😐?	
Bismuth and bismuth compounds (bismuth citrate, bismuth oxychloride etc.; on the NIH HSDB)	Various	☹	
2-Bromo-2-nitropropane 1,3-diol (Bronopol, BNPD; on the Canadian Hotlist)	Preservative Solvent	☹	
5-Bromo-5-nitro-1, 3- dioxane (Bronidox L; on the Canadian Hotlist)	Preservative	☹	
Bronidox L (5-Bromo-5-nitro-1, 3- dioxane)	Preservative	☹	
Bronopol (2-Bromo-2-nitropropane 1,3-diol)	Preservative	☹	
Butyl myristate (from myristic acid and butyl alcohol)	Emollient	☺	

Potential Effects	Cosmetic Uses	Other Uses
Conjunctivitis; eye and skin irritation; contact dermatitis; can be fatal if ingested; toxic	Shampoo, mouthwash, hair conditioner, eye lotion	Antiseptic and detergent in medicinal use
Photosensitivity; skin reactions, especially if skin is dry or sensitive; changes skin pH levels	Skin peels (do not use on infants or children), skin masks, moisturizer	
Adverse effects include memory loss, convulsions, confusion, intellectual impairment; kidney and cardiovascular toxicity	Bleaching and freckle cream, nail polish, hair dye, eye shadow, eye pencil, eyeliner, lipstick	Silvering mirrors, making acrylic fibers, printing industry
Eye and skin irritation; liver toxicity; contact dermatitis; can produce formaldehyde & carcinogenic nitrosamines	Shampoo, mascara, eye makeup, liquid hand wash, nail polish, face cream	
Skin and eye irritation; can release formaldehyde; can form nitrosamines	Shampoo, mascara, eye makeup, liquid hand wash	
See 5-bromo-5-nitro- 1, 3-dioxane	See 5-bromo-5-nitro- 1, 3-dioxane	
See 2-bromo-2-nitropropane-1, 3-diol	See 2-bromo-2-nitropropane-1, 3-diol	
May cause skin irritation; some myristates can promote acne	Lipstick, face cream, nail polish, nail polish remover	

Names	Function	Code
Butylparaben (ester of p-hydroxybenzoic acid & butyl alcohol; on the NIH HSDB)	Preservative	☹
Calcium thioglycolate (synthetic; on the NIH HSDB)	Depilating agent	☹
Caprylic/capric/lauric triglyceride (may be of ANIMAL origin)	Emollient Solvent	☺
Ceresin wax (brittle wax derived from the mineral ozokerite)	Thickener Antistatic agent	☺
Cetalkonium chloride (derived from ammonia)	Preservative Antibacterial	😐?
Cetearyl alcohol (may be natural or synthetic; may be of ANIMAL origin)	Emulsifier Emollient	☺
Cetearyl glucoside (synthetic oleochemical from coconut and corn; may be GE)	Emulsifier	☺
Cetearyl palmitate (may be of ANIMAL origin)	Emollient	☺

Potential Effects	Cosmetic Uses	Other Uses
Allergic and hypersensitivity reactions; skin irritation; see parabens	Cosmetics, shampoo, eye pencil, lipstick, aftershave, baby lotion	Processed foods
Harmful; skin problems on hands or scalp; bleeding under the skin; severe allergic reactions; thyroid problems in animal studies	Hair perm lotion, cream depilatories	Tanning leather, shearing wool
Low toxicity, mild eye and skin irritation	Lipstick, bath oil, soap, perfume, hairspray	
Believed safe in cosmetic use; sensitization in some people	Protective cream, hair conditioner, lipstick, eye pencil, cream blush	Waxed paper and cloth, dentistry
Contact allergies; dry, brittle hair; ingestion can be fatal; see quaternary ammonium compounds	Hair conditioner, deodorant, cosmetics, antiperspirant	
May cause contact dermatitis and contact sensitization in some people	Hair tints, lipstick, shampoo, suntan lotions	
May cause contact dermatitis and contact sensitization in some people	Hand and body lotion, moisturizer	
Some palmitates may cause contact dermatitis	Hand lotion	

Names	Function	Code
Cetrimonium bromide (synthetic)	Preservative	☹
Cetrimonium chloride (synthetic; on the NIH HSDB)	Preservative	😐?
Cetyl alcohol (synthetic oleochemical; may be of plant, ANIMAL, or petrochemical origin; on the NIH HSDB)	Emollient Emulsifier Opacifier	☺
Cetyl palmitate (may be synthetic; may be of ANIMAL origin)	Emollient	☺
Cetyl ricinoleate (may be of ANIMAL origin)	Emollient Solvent	☺
Cetyl stearate (may be synthetic; may be of ANIMAL origin)	Emollient	☺
Chloracetamide (synthetic)	Preservative	😐?
Chlorhexidine (synthetic; on the Canadian Hotlist)	Preservative Topical antiseptic	☹

Potential Effects	Cosmetic Uses	Other Uses
Ingestion can be fatal; can cause skin and eye irritation; reproductive effects; toxic to mice embryos; suspected teratogen	Shampoo, deodorant, skin cleaning products, hair conditioner	
See quaternary ammonium compounds; bioaccumulates in aquatic organisms	Shampoo, hair color, hair conditioner	
Believed to have a low toxicity orally and on the skin; may cause hives and contact dermatitis; skin disorders	Baby lotion, mascaras, foundations, deodorant, antiperspirants, hair color, shampoo, hair conditioner	Laxatives
Believed safe in cosmetic use; some palmitates can cause contact dermatitis	Eye makeup, hand and body lotion, shampoo, moisturizer	Manufacture of lubricants
Believed safe in cosmetic use; may cause eye irritation	Suntan lotion, skin cleanser, lipstick	
No known toxicity or adverse reactions	Skin conditioner in cosmetic products	
See quaternary ammonium compounds	Cold cream, mud packs, shampoo, cleansing lotion	
Contact dermatitis; immuno and respiratory toxicity; has been known to cause anaphylactic shock	Liquid cosmetics, feminine hygiene spray, deodorant	

Names	Function	Code
Chlorobutanol (chlorbutanol; acetone chloroform)	Preservative Antioxidant	☹
Chlorothymol (thymol derivative; phenolic compound)	Oral care agent Deodorant	☺?
Coal tar and coal tar dyes (contains creosol, naphthalene, quinoline, xylene, phenol, benzene, and others; on the Canadian Hotlist; banned for general use in the EU; see glossary)	Colorant Antidandruff agent	☹☹
Cocamide DEA (semi-synthetic)	Emulsifier Surfactant	☹
Cocamide MEA (synthetic)	Surfactant Emulsifier	☺?
Cocamidopropyl betaine (synthetic)	Surfactant	☺?
Cocoa butter (theobroma oil; from roasted seeds of the cocoa plant)	Emollient Emulsifier	☺

Potential Effects	Cosmetic Uses	Other Uses
Acute oral toxicity; allergic reactions; CNS depression; harmful if inhaled; can be absorbed into the skin	Eye lotion, baby oil	Treating mastitis in cows
Can cause skin rash and mucous membrane irritation if combined with chlorine; can be absorbed via the skin	Mouthwash, hair tonic, baby oil	Topical antibacterial medication
Contact dermatitis; hives; respiratory and skin toxicity; psoriasis; phototoxicity; acne; skin rash; breast, bladder and liver cancers; harmful to the environment	Shampoo, hair dye, facial cosmetics, hand and body lotion, toothpastes	Adhesives, insecticides, creosotes, phenols
Allergic skin rash; can contain DEA; see diethanolamine	Shampoo, bubble bath, shaving gel, moisturizer	Pet shampoo
Mild skin reactions in some people; vapor is highly toxic; may contain nitrosamines; harmful to the environment	Shampoo, body wash, hair conditioner	Pet shampoo, toilet bowl cleaner
Contact dermatitis; allergic reactions; eyelid rash	Soap, eye makeup remover, shampoo	
Softens and lubricates the skin; may cause allergic skin reactions and cosmetic acne	Blush, nail whitener, lipstick, hand and body lotion	Sweet sauces, candy, suppositories

Names	Function	Code
Coco-betaine (synthetic; from coconut oil)	Surfactant	☺
Coconut oil (from coconut kernels; on the NIH HSDB)	Surfactant Emollient Solvent	☺
Crystalline silica	Colorant Abrasive	☹
D & C colors; e.g. D & C red no. 6 (blue, brown, green, red, orange, violet and yellow)	Colorant	☺?
DEA and DEA compounds (diethanolamine)	Solvent Emulsifier	☹
Decyl alcohol (derived from liquid paraffin)	Antifoaming agent Fixative	☺
Decyl myristate (may be of ANIMAL origin)	Emollient	☺
Decyl oleate (may be of ANIMAL origin)	Emollient Emulsifier	☺
Decyl polyglucose (decyl alcohol and glucose)	Surfactant	☺
2,4-Diaminoanisole (synthetic)	Colorant	☹

Potential Effects	Cosmetic Uses	Other Uses
May cause skin rash in sensitive people	Shampoo, face and hand gel	
May alleviate dry skin; may cause allergic skin rashes; eye and skin irritation	Shampoo, baby soap, massage cream, hair gel	Margarine, car polish, cigarettes
Eye, skin and lung irritation when used in its dry form; carcinogenic	Blusher, lip pencils, facial powder	Cat litter, cleanser, paint, floor adhesive
Most can cause health effects including skin rash, allergic reactions, asthma	Most cosmetics, including soap, lip gloss, nail polish	
See diethanolamine	See diethanolamine	
Believed safe in cosmetic use; low toxicity on the skin in animal testing	Cosmetics, perfume	Fruit flavoring in foods
Myristates can promote acne in some people	Skin conditioner in cosmetics	
May promote acne in some people; safety under review	Hand cream, suntan products	
May cause skin irritation in sensitive people	Shampoo, liquid hand soap, body wash	
Allergic contact dermatitis; suspected mutagen and recognized carcinogen	Hair dye	

Names	Function	Code	
2,4-Diaminophenol (synthetic)	Colorant	☹	
Diazolidinyl urea (Germall II; of ANIMAL origin)	Preservative	☹	
Dibromofluorescein (made by heating resorcinol with a naphthalene derivative)	Colorant	☹	
Dichlorophene (crystals from toluene)	Anti-microbial	☹	
Diethanolamine (DEA; from ethylene oxide, ammonia and ethanolamines; on the NIH HSDB, see nitrosamines)	Solvent Buffer	☹	

Potential Effects	Cosmetic Uses	Other Uses
See phenylenediamine	Hair dye	
Sensitizer; eye and skin irritation; contact dermatitis; may release formaldehyde; not readily biodegradable	Shampoo, mascara, hair conditioner, shaving gel, moisturizer	Pesticides, textile industry, pet shampoo
Skin and eye inflammation; skin rash; respiratory and gastrointestinal symptoms; sensitivity to light	Indelible lipstick	
Harmful; developmental and neurotoxicity; skin rashes; allergic reactions	Shampoo, antiperspirant, deodorant	
Hormone disruption; mucous membrane & skin irritation; cardiovascular, kidney, liver, gastrointestinal and neurotoxicity; can combine with nitrosating agents to form NDELA, a carcinogenic nitrosamine; may be toxic to aquatic organisms	Soap, bubble bath, hair conditioner, moisturizing cream, liquid hand soap, shampoo. Should not be used in products that contain nitrosating agents.	Car wash detergent, cutting oils, cleaners, polishes

Names	Function	Code	
Diethyl phthalate (made from ethanol and benzene derivatives)	Solvent Fixative Denaturant	☹☹	
Diethylene glycol (by-product of ethylene glycol production; concentrations over 10% hazardous; on the NIH HSDB)	Humectant Solvent	☹☹	
Dihexyl adipate (from adipic acid; see adipic acid in section 1)	Emollient Solvent	☺	
Diisopropanolamine (on the NIH HSDB)	Acid-alkali adjuster Emulsifier	☺?	
1,4-Dioxane (created during the manufacturing process; can be removed from products by vacuum stripping; on the Canadian Hotlist)	Contaminant	☹	

Potential Effects	Cosmetic Uses	Other Uses
CNS depression; mucous membrane irritation; skin, liver, endocrine, respiratory and neurotoxicity; suspected teratogen; environmental hazard; bioaccumulates in aquatic organisms	Perfume, nail polish, moisturizer	Insect repellant, food packaging, varnish
Ingestion can be fatal; skin and eye irritation; kidney, blood, liver & neurotoxicity; suspected teratogen	Cosmetic cream, hairspray	Cartridge inks, paint, paracetamol elixirs
Adipic acid has no known human toxicity but large oral doses are lethal to rats	Moisturizer, skin care products, makeup	
Can combine with nitrosating agents to form nitrosamines	Hair dye, perms, hair grooming aids	Polishes, insecticides, cutting oils
Cardiovascular, respiratory, gastrointestinal, immuno, endocrine, kidney, liver and neurotoxicity; suspected mutagen and teratogen; recognized carcinogen	May be present in processed foods, chlorine bleached paper, plastic lined cartons and cans	Adhesive, released when plastic is burnt, newsprint, pesticides

Names	Function	Code
Dioxins (TCDD is one of the most hazardous; a by-product of the herbicide Agent Orange; highly toxic and carcinogenic contaminants; on the Canadian Hotlist)	Contaminant	☹☹
Distearyldimonium chloride (on the NIH HSDB)	Antistatic agent	😐?
DMDM hydantoin (derived from methanol)	Preservative	☹
Drometrizole (derived from benzene)	Solvent UV absorber	☹
Elastin (may be of ANIMAL origin)	Biological additive	☺
Ethanolamines (mono, di and tri-forms)	Preservative Emulsifier	☹

Potential Effects	Cosmetic Uses	Other Uses
Cardiovascular, respiratory, developmental, liver, kidney, gastrointestinal, endocrine, reproductive, immuno and neurotoxicity; behavioral and learning problems; mutagenic; teratogenic; carcinogenic	May be present in processed foods, chlorine bleached paper, plastic lined cartons and cans	Released when plastic is burnt, newsprint, pesticides
See quaternary ammonium compounds	Moisturizer, baby lotion, shampoo, hair rinse	Fabric softener
Skin and eye irritation; allergic reactions; dermatitis; may release formaldehyde	Cosmetics, shampoo, mascara, cream conditioner	Dishwashing liquid, metal polish
Determined not to be safe in cosmetic use by CIR Expert Panel; see benzene	Nail polish, cosmetics	
Believed safe in cosmetic use; may coat the skin inhibiting proper function	Shampoo, hair conditioner, skin cream and lotion	
Irritating to lungs, skin and eyes; hair loss; sensitization; may be contaminated with carcinogenic nitrosamines	Hair dye, perms, soap	

Names	Function	Code
Ethoxyethanol (from ethylene chloride, sodium acetate and alcohol; on the Canadian Hotlist)	Solvent	☹
Ethylenediamine (synthetic; on the Canadian Hotlist)	Solvent pH control	☹
Ethylene glycol (prepared from ethylene oxide; on the NIH HSDB)	Solvent	☹
Ethyl methacrylate (ester of ethyl alcohol and methacrylic acid; on the Canadian Hotlist)	Thickening agents	☹
Ethylparaben (from p-hydroxybenzoic acid and ethanol; on the NIH HSDB)	Preservative	☹
Fluorescein (synthetic)	Coloring	☹

Potential Effects	Cosmetic Uses	Other Uses
CNS depression; kidney damage; developmental and reproductive toxicity; can penetrate unbroken skin	Cosmetics, nail polish, shampoo	
Toxic if inhaled or absorbed by the skin; severe skin and eye irritation; sensitization; asthma; contact dermatitis; toxic to aquatic organisms	Thigh cream, cosmetics	Metal polish, pesticides
CNS depression; immuno, respiratory, gastrointestinal, liver, kidney & neurotoxicity; contact dermatitis	Perfume, liquid soap, cosmetics	Insect repellant, antifreeze, car wax, shoe products
Skin irritation; allergic reactions; neurotoxicity; allergic contact dermatitis; suspected teratogen; AVOID SKIN CONTACT	Nail polish, artificial nails	
Contact dermatitis; allergic & hypersensitivity reactions; skin irritation; see parabens	Cosmetics, makeup, shampoo, deodorant, mascara	Pharmaceuticals
Photosensitivity; respiratory and gastrointestinal symptoms; lip inflammation	Indelible lipstick, nail polish	Dying wool, silk and paper

Names	Function	Code
Fluoride (byproduct of aluminum and fertilizer manufacture; cumulative poison; classified as a contaminant by the USEPA; on the Canadian Hotlist; on the NIH HSDB)	Oral care Preservative Insecticide	☹😧
Geranium oil (extract from plants)	Botanical additive	😐?
Glutaraldehyde (glutaral; synthetic; on the NIH HSDB)	Preservative Germicide	☹😧
Glyceryl myristate (may be of ANIMAL origin)	Emulsifier Stabilizer	😐?
Glyceryl stearate (may be of ANIMAL origin)	Emulsifier Emollient	😐?

Potential Effects	Cosmetic Uses	Other Uses
Hypothyroidism; arthritis; osteoporosis; carpal tunnel syndrome; impaired brain function; birth defects; hip fractures; stress fractures; kidney, musculoskeletal, liver & neurotoxicity; skeletal & dental fluorosis; suspected bone cancer; teratogen	Toothpaste, cosmetics, mouthwash, dentifrices	Many products containing water e.g. soft drinks, cordial, fruit juice, canned & bottled foods, public water supplies, dental treatments
Contact dermatitis and skin irritation in some people; ingestion can be fatal	Tooth powder, dusting powder, foundation, perfume	Ointments
Contact allergic reactions; contact dermatitis; nausea; headache; aches and pains; palpitations; mood swings; asthma; developmental, respiratory, reproductive, skin and immunotoxicity; suspected teratogen; very toxic to aquatic organisms	Antiperspirant, hairspray, deodorant, setting lotion, waterless hand soap	Food flavoring; disinfectant used in hospitals and dentistry, biocide in cosmetics and the oil industry, embalming fluid
May promote acne; may cause contact dermatitis	Baby cream, face masks, hand lotion	
May cause skin allergies and contact dermatitis	Makeup, mascara, baby lotion, cuticle softener	

Names	Function	Code	
Glyceryl thioglycolate	Depilatory agent Reducing agent	☹	
Glycolic acid (made synthetically from chloroacetic acid; see also alpha hydroxy acids)	Buffer Exfoliant	☺?	
Guar hydroxypropyltrimonium chloride	Antistatic agent	☺?	
Henna extract (from the ground-up dried leaves and stems of a shrub)	Colorant (red)	☺	
Hexachlorophene (prohibited in most cosmetic products in the EU and USA; on the Canadian Hotlist)	Preservative	☹☹	
Hexylene glycol (synthetic; from the hydrogenation of diacetone alcohol; on the NIH HSDB)	Solvent Viscosity controlling agent	☹	

Potential Effects	Cosmetic Uses	Other Uses
Thioglycolates can cause skin irritations, contact dermatitis, severe allergic reactions and hair breakage	Hair perms, depilatories	
Mildly irritating to skin and mucous membranes; may cause sun sensitivity; exfoliative dermatitis	Skin peels (do not use on infants or children)	Dyeing, brightening copper
See quaternary ammonium compounds	Shampoo, body wash, hair conditioner	
One of the safest hair dyes; rarely causes allergic skin rash, avoid use near eyes	Hair dye, hair conditioner and rinse, shampoo	
Multiple sclerosis; contact dermatitis; gastrointestinal, liver and neurotoxicity; birth defects; asthma; blindness; chloasma; allergic reactions; toxic to aquatic organisms; bioaccumulates in the food chain e.g. milk; long term environmental effects	Antiperspirant, deodorant, baby oil, shampoo, toothpaste, cold cream, baby powder	Washing fruit, detergents, animal products
Contact dermatitis; eye, skin and mucous membrane irritation; gastrointestinal, liver, respiratory and neurotoxicity	Cleansing lotion, hair color, moisturizer, hair conditioner	Toilet bowel cleaner, fabric softener, brake fluid, printing ink

Names	Function	Code
Homosalate (homomethyl salicylate)	UV absorber	☺?
Hydroquinone (synthetic; from aniline or quinone; on the Canadian Hotlist; on the NIH HSDB)	Antioxidant Bleaching agent	☹☹
Hydroxyanisole (p-hydroxyanisole; derived from hardwood tar or made synthetically; on the Canadian Hotlist)	Antioxidant	☹
Hydroxyethylcellulose (from cellulose by petrochemicals; may be GE; on the NIH HSDB)	Binder Film former	☺
Hydroxymethylglycinate	Preservative	☺?
Hydroxymethylcellulose	Thickener Additive	☺
Imidazolidinyl urea (of ANIMAL origin)	Preservative	☹

Potential Effects	Cosmetic Uses	Other Uses
Endocrine disruption; reports of poisonings when absorbed through the skin	Sunscreen	
Nausea, vomiting, delirium and collapse from ingestion; eye damage; contact allergy; contact dermatitis; liver and neurotoxicity; sensitization; animal carcinogen; very toxic to aquatic organisms	Freckle cream, suntan lotion, hair coloring, shampoo	Super glue, fats and oils, paints, varnishes, dyes, motor oils and fuels, developer in photography
Non-Hodgkin's lymphoma; skin de-pigmentation; eye and skin irritation; ingestion can cause intestinal tract irritation and heart failure	Permanent hair color, lipstick	
Believed safe in cosmetic use; adverse reactions are rare	Shampoo, tanning, products, mascara, hand and body lotion	Toilet bowl cleaner
May release formaldehyde; see formaldehyde in Section 1	Cosmetics	
Believed safe in cosmetic use; adverse reactions rare	Cosmetics, hair care products	
Contact dermatitis; may release formaldehyde; see formaldehyde	Baby shampoo, eye makeup, bath oil, moisturizer, blush	

Names	Function	Code	
Isopropyl isostearate (may be of ANIMAL origin)	Emollient	☺	
Isopropyl lanolate (of ANIMAL origin)	Lubricant Emollient	☺?	
Isopropyl myristate (may be of ANIMAL origin; on the NIH HSDB)	Moisturizer Emollient Solvent	☺?	
Isopropyl palmitate (may be of ANIMAL origin; on the NIH HSDB)	Emollient Preservative	☺?	
Isopropyl stearate (may be of ANIMAL origin)	Emollient Binder	☺?	
Isostearyl palmitate (may be of ANIMAL origin)	Surfactant Emollient	☺	
Japan wax (from the fruit of trees grown in China and Japan)	Emulsifier	☺?	
Kaolin (China clay; hydrated aluminum silicate; on the NIH HSDB)	Anti-caking agent Absorbent	☺?	

Potential Effects	Cosmetic Uses	Other Uses
Believed safe in cosmetic use; may promote acne; skin irritation when undiluted	Skin conditioner, skin cleanser, eye shadow, lipstick, moisturizer	
Skin sensitization; safety is under review	Bath gel, skin cream, lipstick	
May significantly increase the absorption of NDELA, a carcinogenic contaminant found in some cosmetics; may promote acne	Suntan lotion, bath oil, shampoo, hand lotion, deodorant	Pesticides
Eye and skin irritation; allergic reactions	Moisturizer, baby lotion, cologne, shampoo, hand and body lotion	Pesticides
May cause skin irritation and allergic reactions	Skin conditioner, hair remover	Pesticides
May be a sensitizer for those who suffer allergies; may cause contact dermatitis	Hand cream, shaving cream, soap, protective cream, cleansing lotion	
Allergic contact dermatitis	Eyeliner, eye pencils	
May inhibit proper skin function by clogging pores; chronic inhalation can affect the lungs leading to fibrosis	Baby powder, bath powder, face powder, makeup, mascara, hair conditioner	Metal polish, beer production, making pottery, porcelain, bricks

Names	Function	Code
Kathon CG (on the Canadian Hotlist; on the NIH HSDB)	Preservative	☹
Lanolin; lanolin oil; lanolin wax (wool fat; may be contaminated with pesticides; of ANIMAL origin; on the NIH HSDB)	Emulsifier Emollient	☺?
Lauramide DEA (synthetic derivative of coconut oil; on the NIH HSDB)	Thickener Foam booster	☹
Lauramide MEA (synthetic derivative of coconut oil; on the NIH HSDB)	Antistatic agent	☺?
Lauroyl lysine (may be of ANIMAL origin)	Viscosity controlling agent	☺☺
Lauryl alcohol (derived from coconut oil; on the NIH HSDB)	Surfactant Emollient	☺?
Lavender extract and oil (from the fresh flowery tops of the lavender plant)	Fragrance	☺
Linoleamide DEA (diethanolamine and linoleic acid)	Foaming agent Antistatic agent	☹

Potential Effects	Cosmetic Uses	Other Uses
Contact dermatitis; potent sensitizer; bacterial mutagen; skin cancer	Shampoo, cosmetics	Leather preservation
Believed to be safe if uncontaminated; may cause allergic skin reactions, acne and contact dermatitis	Lipstick, mascara, nail polish remover, eye makeup, hair conditioner	Pesticides
Itchy scalp; allergic skin reactions; dry hair; may contain DEA; see diethanolamine	Shampoo, liquid soap, hair conditioner, bubble bath	Dishwashing detergent, pet shampoo
May cause mild skin irritation; may contain DEA; see diethanolamine	Shampoo, hair color, hair conditioner	Dishwashing detergent, pet shampoo
Believed safe in cosmetic use	Facial powder, lipstick, eye shadow, makeup	
Skin irritation; may promote acne	Perfume, shampoo, body wash, shave gel	Detergents
Believed to have beneficial effects on health; may cause allergic contact dermatitis; photosensitivity?	Shampoo, baby oil, skin fresheners, mouthwash, perfume, dentifrices	Antiseptic oils, cream and lotion, cigarettes
Can contain DEA; see diethanolamine	Shampoo	

Names	Function	Code	
Linoleamide MEA (mixture of ethanolamides of linoleic acid)	Surfactant Antistatic agent	☺?	
Mercury and mercury compounds (quicksilver; prohibited in most cosmetic products in the USA; on the Canadian Hotlist; on the NIH HSDB)	Preservative	☹☹	
Methacrylic acid (synthetic; on the Canadian Hotlist; on the NIH HSDB)	Primer	☹	
Methenamine (made from formaldehyde and ammonia; on the NIH HSDB)	Preservative Antiseptic	☹	
Methoxyethanol (ethylene glycol ether; on the NIH HSDB; on the Canadian Hotlist)	Solvent Fragrance	☹	
5-Methoxypsoralen (5-MOP; banned from cosmetics in the EU)	UV absorber	☹	
8-Methoxypsoralen (methoxysalen)	UV absorber	☹	

Potential Effects	Cosmetic Uses	Other Uses
May be irritating to the skin and eyes; may contain DEA; see diethanolamine	Eye cream, hair care products	
Extremely toxic; respiratory, reproductive, blood, liver, kidney and neurotoxicity; autism; epilepsy; suspected teratogen; can be absorbed through the skin; very toxic to aquatic organisms	Medicated soap, cosmetics, freckle cream, face masks, hair tonic	Dyes, paint, fungicides, plastics
Poisonous if ingested; skin and nail damage; burns; inflammation; infection; neurotoxicity	Artificial nail kits; nail products	Adhesives, resins, hydrogel contact lenses, plastics
Can release formaldehyde; nitrosamine precursor; skin irritation; skin rash	Hair conditioner, shampoo	Medicines
Birth defects; developmental and reproductive toxicity	Nail polish, perfume, liquid soap, cosmetics	
Increased risk of skin cancer; contact allergy; photoallergy; neurotoxicity; recognized carcinogen	Suntan accelerator, sunscreen	
See methoxysalen	See methoxysalen	

Names	Function	Code	
Methoxysalen (8-MOP; banned from cosmetics in the EU)	UV absorber	☹	
Methylchloroisothiazolinone (on the Canadian Hotlist)	Preservative	☺?	
Methyldibromoglutaronitrile (synthetic)	Preservative	☹	
Methylisothiazolinone (on the Canadian Hotlist)	Preservative	☺?	
Methyl methacrylate (banned in the EU; on the Canadian Hotlist)	Film former	☹☹	
Methylparaben (methyl p-hydroxybenzoate)	Preservative	☹	

Potential Effects	Cosmetic Uses	Other Uses
Contact allergy; liver, skin & neurotoxicity; photoallergy; recognized carcinogen	Suntan accelerator, sunscreen	
Allergic reactions; contact dermatitis; may be mutagenic	Shampoo, liquid hand and body wash, bubble bath, aftershave	Dishwashing liquid, shoe cleaner, paint
Believed unsafe for use in cosmetic products; allergic reactions; contact dermatitis; skin sensitization	Hair conditioner, bubble bath, self-tanners, shampoo, body soap	Dishwashing liquid
See methylchloro-isothiazolinone	Body wash, shampoo, hair conditioner	Shoe cleaner, pet shampoo, paint
Severe skin irritation; contact dermatitis; allergic reactions; gastrointestinal, reproductive, liver, blood, respiratory, kidney, immuno and neurotoxicity; suspected teratogen; toxic to aquatic organisms	Nail polish, artificial nails	Medical and dental orthopedic cement, adhesives
May cause allergic reactions; contact dermatitis; see parabens	Many cosmetic and personal care products	Pet shampoo

Names	Function	Code
Mexenone (2-Hydroxy-4-methoxy- 4'-methyl-benzophenone)	UV absorber	😐?
Mica (pulverized silicate minerals; on the NIH HSDB)	Opacifier Colorant	😊?
Monoethanolamine (MEA & ingredients ending in MEA; from ammonia and ethylene oxide or nitromethane and formaldehyde; on the NIH HSDB)	Humectant Emulsifier	😐?
Montan wax (derived from lignite)	Emulsifier	😊
2-Naphthol (beta-naphthol; from naphthalene from coal tar; on the Canadian Hotlist)	Solvent Modifier	😖😖
Neem seed oil (from a tree native to India)	Antibacterial Antiviral	😊
Neomycin (antibiotic; antibiotics are banned from cosmetics in the EU	Antibiotic	😖

Potential Effects	Cosmetic Uses	Other Uses
Photoallergy; hives; contact allergy; chronic actinic dermatitis; can mimic or exacerbate an illness; see benzophenones in section 1	Sunscreen	
May cause irritation and lung damage if powder inhaled; gastrointestinal and liver toxicity	Face powder, eye makeup, lipstick, shampoo, mascara, foundation	Cat litter
Can cause skin and eye irritation; may cause carcinogenic nitrosamine formation	Shampoo, hand cleaner, body lotion, hair color, skin cleanser, liquid soap	Oven cleaner, laundry detergent, paint stripper, degreaser
Believed non-toxic in cosmetic uses	Lipstick, foundations	
Kidney damage, eye injury, convulsions, anemia and death from ingestion; skin damage; contact dermatitis	Hair products, hair dye, skin peels, perfume	Manufacture of agrochemicals
Believed to relieve dry skin, eczema, acne and dandruff; teratogen?	Skin cream, soap, lipstick, shampoo	Insect repellant
Can cause allergic reactions, photoallergy, kidney toxicity, may promote staphylococcus infections	May be used in some underarm deodorant	

Names	Function	Code	
Nickel sulfate (synthetic)	Additive	☹	
Nitrites (sodium, potassium etc.)	Preservative Color fixative	☹☹	
Nitrobenzene (essence of mirabane; nitric acid and benzene; on the Canadian Hotlist)	Fragrance Solvent	☹☹	
2-Nitro-p-phenylenediamine (derived from coal tar)	Colorant	☹☹	
Nitrosamines (toxic group of compounds formed when nitrites and nitrates combine with amines; e.g. NDELA may be found in cosmetics and shampoo; on the Canadian Hotlist)	Contaminant	☹☹	
Octyl dimethyl PABA (Padamate O; on the NIH HSDB)	UV absorber	☹	

Potential Effects	Cosmetic Uses	Other Uses
Skin rash; kidney, endocrine & immunotoxicity; vomiting if ingested; contact dermatitis	Hair dye, eye pencils, cosmetics, astringents	Dietary supplement, nickel plating
May combine with amines found in the stomach, saliva, foods and cosmetics to form carcinogenic nitrosamines	Sodium nitrite is used as an anticorrosive in some cosmetics	Cured meats, matches, tobacco
Absorbed through the skin; reproductive, respiratory, gastrointestinal, kidney, liver and neurotoxicity; nausea; headache; drowsiness; suspected teratogen	Cheap scented soaps	Making aniline a base for dye and drugs, shoe polish
See phenylenediamine	Permanent and semi-permanent hair dye	Dyeing furs
Implicated in many forms of cancer including liver, lung, mouth, stomach and esophageal; liver damage; can pass through the skin; environmental effects not adequately investigated	Cosmetic products and shampoo with DEA, MEA or TEA compounds unless removed by the manufacturer	Found in air, tobacco smoke, pesticides, water, cured meats
See amyl dimethyl PABA	See amyl dimethyl PABA	

Names	Function	Code	
Octyl methoxycinnamate (synthetic)	UV absorber	☺?	
Octyl palmitate (may be of ANIMAL origin)	Emollient	☺	
Oleic acid (may be of ANIMAL origin; on the NIH HSDB)	Emollient De-foaming agent	☺	
Oleoyl sarcosine (may be of ANIMAL origin)	Antistatic agent Surfactant	☺?	
Oxybenzone (derived from isopropanol)	UV absorber	☺?	
Padimate A (amyl dimethyl PABA)	UV absorber	☹	
Padimate O (octyl dimethyl PABA)	UV absorber	☹	
Parabens (butyl, ethyl, methyl, propyl etc; synthetic; esters of hydroxybenzoic acid)	Preservative	☹	

Potential Effects	Cosmetic Uses	Other Uses
Photoallergy and contact allergy; endocrine disruption	Sunscreen, lipstick, perfume, foundation	Insect repellant
Believed safe in cosmetic use; may cause cosmetic acne	Cold cream, shaving cream, moisturizer, lipstick	
Low oral toxicity; may cause mild skin and eye irritation; may promote acne	Soft soap, lipstick, baby lotion, shampoo, hair color, mascara	Cigarettes
Can cause mild skin irritation; sarcosines can enhance absorption of other ingredients through the skin and can cause nitrosamine contamination	Soap, cosmetics, lubricants, hair conditioner	Polishing compounds
Photosensitivity; chronic actinic dermatitis; contact allergy	Sunscreen	
See amyl dimethyl PABA	Sunscreen	
See octyl dimethyl PABA	Makeup, sunscreen	
Allergic reactions; endocrine disruption; contact dermatitis; may increase the risk of breast cancer; toxic in animals by ingestion	Many cosmetic and personal care products	Various processed foods

Names	Function	Code	
Phenoxyethanol (2-phenoxyethanol; derived from phenol and ethylene oxide; on the NIH HSDB)	Solvent Fixative Preservative	☺?	
Phenylenediamine (m-, o-, p-) (on the Canadian Hotlist; p form is on the NIH HSDB)	Colorant	☹☹	
Phenyl mercuric acetate (contains mercury)	Preservative Fungicide	☹☹	
Polyethylene (may be contaminated with the carcinogen 1,4- dioxane)	Binder Antistatic Stabilizer	☺?	
Polyoxyethylene compounds (may be contaminated with the carcinogen 1,4- dioxane)	Emulsifier	☺?	

Potential Effects	Cosmetic Uses	Other Uses
Inhalation or skin contact can cause nausea, diarrhea, headache, CNS depression, vomiting and renal failure	Shampoo, cleansing cream, perfume, hair color, lipstick, mascara	Insect repellant, antifreeze, dyes, inks, filler in vaccines
Contact dermatitis; asthma; blindness; photoallergy; skin, cardiovascular, kidney, immuno and neurotoxicity; animal carcinogen; can be absorbed via the skin; very toxic to aquatic organisms	Most home and beauty salon hair dyes, eyelash dyes	
Very toxic internally; skin irritation; allergic reactions; toxic to aquatic organisms; bioaccumulates in the food chain e.g. water organisms, fish, crustacea, birds	Eye makeup and eye makeup remover, shampoo	Paint
No known skin toxicity; large doses caused cancer in rats; ingestion of large doses can cause liver & kidney damage	Hand lotion, mascara, skin fresheners, suntan products, underarm deodorant	Chewing gum, sheets for packaging
Sensitivity reactions; eye and skin irritation	Hand cream, hand lotion	Air freshener

Names	Function	Code
Potassium chlorate (synthetic)	Oxidizing agent	☹
Psoralen (derived from a plant)	UV absorber	😐?
Pycnogenol (blend of bioflavonoids)	Antioxidant	☺☺
Pyrocatechol (coal tar derivative; on the Canadian Hotlist)	Antiseptic Oxidizer	☹
Pyrogallol (a phenol; on the Canadian Hotlist)	Antiseptic Colorant	☹
Quaternary ammonium compounds (QUATS; synthetic derivatives of ammonium chloride)	Various	😐?
Quaternium-15 (may break down to, or release formaldehyde; on the NIH HSDB)	Preservative	☹

Potential Effects	Cosmetic Uses	Other Uses
Gum inflammation; dermatitis; intestinal and kidney irritation; may be absorbed through the skin	Toothpaste, freckle lotion, mouthwash, gargle	Bleach, fireworks, pesticides, matches
Photodermatitis; photosensitivity	Sunscreen, perfume	Treatment of vitiligo
Believed to have beneficial effects on health	Anti-aging products	Chewing gum, dietary supplements
Contact dermatitis, eczema; kidney and liver toxicity; suspected carcinogen	Hair dye (blonde), skin care preparations	Photography, dyeing furs
Skin sensitization; ingestion can cause kidney and liver damage; suspected mutagen and teratogen; toxic to aquatic organisms	Permanent hair dye, skin care preparations	Anti-microbial, used medically to soothe irritated skin
Depending on concentration and dose all QUATS can be toxic; contact dermatitis; eye and mucous membrane irritation; anaphylaxis (rare)	Aerosol deodorant, antiperspirant, hand cream, mouthwash, shampoo, lipstick, aftershave lotion	Medical sterilization of mucous membranes, all-purpose cleaner
Contact dermatitis; allergic reactions; eye irritation; skin rash; sensitization	Cosmetics, shampoo, hair conditioner, baby oil, eye shadow	Pet shampoo

Names	Function	Code	
Quaternium-26 (may be contaminated with pesticides and DEA)	Surfactant Antistatic agent	☹	
Quaternium-18 hectorite	Viscosity controller	☺?	
Quercetin (type of bioflavonoid; on the NIH HSDB)	Colorant Antioxidant	☺	
Resorcinol (derived from resins or may be synthetic; on the NIH HSDB)	Preservative Antiseptic Colorant	☹	
Retinol (Vitamin A; may be of ANIMAL origin; on the Canadian Hotlist)	Preservative Additive	☺	
Retinyl palmitate (ester of vitamin A; may be of ANIMAL origin; on the Canadian Hotlist)	Texturiser Additive	☺	

Potential Effects	Cosmetic Uses	Other Uses
Eye irritation; contact dermatitis; suspected carcinogen; see diethanolamine (DEA)	Products giving sheen to hair	
See quaternary ammonium compounds and hectorite	Mascara, suntan gels, moisturizer, lip color	
Believed to have beneficial health effects; may cause allergic reactions; suspected teratogen	Dark brown shades of hair dye	Food additives, dyeing artificial hairpieces, dietary supplements
Eye and eyelid inflammation; dizziness; restlessness; endocrine disruption; liver, immuno, cardiovascular and neurotoxicity; toxic to aquatic organisms	Antidandruff shampoo, hair dye, lipstick, permanent hair color	Tanning, explosives, printing textiles
Believed to have beneficial health effects; excess levels can cause yellow skin, birth defects and liver toxicity	Massage cream and oils, skin care preparations, moisturizer, hand cream, anti-wrinkle treatment	Topical acne treatments
Believed to have beneficial health effects; safe in cosmetic use up to 1% concentration; contact dermatitis	Shampoo, lipstick, body wash, shaving cream; makeup; hand and body lotion, suntan products, hair conditioner	

Names	Function	Code
Ricinoleic acid (from castor beans; on the NIH HSDB)	Emollient Emulsifier	😐?
Rose hips oil (from rose hips)	Botanical additive	😊😊
Rosin (obtained from pine trees)	Viscosity control	😐?
Safrole (toxic component of some natural volatile oils; on the Canadian Hotlist; on the NIH HSDB)	Fragrance	😞😞
Sarcosines and sarcosinates (found in starfish and sea urchins or formed from caffeine; may be of ANIMAL origin)	Surfactant	😐?
Selenium sulfide (on the Canadian Hotlist; on the NIH HSDB)	Antidandruff agent	😞
Shea butter (from fruit of the karite tree)	Emollient Emulsifier	😊😊
Silver nitrate (synthetic)	Colorant	😞

Potential Effects	Cosmetic Uses	Other Uses
Allergic reactions; dermatitis	Soap, lipstick	Contraceptive jelly
Believed to have beneficial effects on the skin	Skin cream, sun care products	
May cause contact allergies; eyelid dermatitis; asthma	Soap, mascara, wax depilatories	Chewing gum, varnishes
Kidney, gastrointestinal, liver, reproductive and neurotoxicity; recognized carcinogen; suspected teratogen	Cheap soaps and perfumes	Manufacture of the flavoring chemical heliotropin
Non-irritating and non-sensitizing; can cause formation of nitrosamines; can enhance penetration of other ingredients through the skin; see nitrosamines	Shampoo, dentifrices, soap, lubricating oils	Dishwashing liquids
Skin irritation; dryness of hair and scalp; liver and musculoskeletal toxicity; severe eye irritation; recognized carcinogen	Medicated antidandruff shampoo	Treatment for tinea versicolor
Softens and moisturizes skin; no known toxicity	Moisturizer, lipstick, lip balm, suntan gel	
Poisonous; caustic and irritating; skin sensitivity; allergies; very toxic to aquatic organisms	Metallic hair dye	

Names	Function	Code	
SLES (sodium laureth sulfate)	Surfactant Detergent	☹	
SLS (sodium lauryl sulfate)	Surfactant Emulsifier	☹	
Sodium alpha-olefin sulfonates (synthetic)	Cleanser	☺?	
Sodium cocoyl isethionate (synthetic)	Surfactant	☺	
Sodium cocoyl sarcosinate (may be of ANIMAL origin)	Surfactant	☺?	
Sodium fluoride (on the Canadian Hotlist; on the NIH HSDB; see also fluoride)	Preservative Oral care agent	☹☹	
Sodium hydroxymethylglycinate (contains formaldehyde as a preservative)	Preservative	☺?	
Sodium laureth sulfate (may contain carcinogens 1,4-dioxane and ethylene oxide; on the NIH HSDB)	Surfactant Detergent	☹	

Potential Effects	Cosmetic Uses	Other Uses
See sodium laureth sulfate	See sodium laureth sulfate	See sodium laureth sulfate
See sodium lauryl sulfate	See sodium lauryl sulfate	See sodium lauryl sulfate
May cause eye and skin irritation & sensitization; fetal abnormalities in animals	Shampoo, bath and shower products	
Believed safe in cosmetic use; mild skin and eye irritation	Bar soap, body wash, moisturizer, mousse	
See sarcosines	Skin cleanser, hand and body wash	
Brittle bones; joint stiffness; discolored tooth enamel; gastrointestinal, respiratory, developmental, liver, skin cardiovascular and neurotoxicity	Mouthwash, toothpaste, dentifrices	Cigarettes
May release formaldehyde; the NIH could not locate any studies for safety	Hair conditioner, hair gel, baby wipes, personal cleansing wipes	
Mild eye and skin irritation; can cause the formation of nitrosamines; toxic to aquatic organisms; see nitrosamines	Shampoo, toothpaste, bath gel, bubble bath, liquid hand and body wash, mascara, liquid hand soap	Dishwashing liquid, laundry detergent

Names	Function	Code
Sodium lauryl sulfate (synthetic, by sulfation of lauryl alcohol and neutralization with sodium carbonate or sodium hydroxide; on the NIH HSDB)	Surfactant Emulsifier	☹
Sodium lauryl sulfoacetate (synthetic)	Surfactant	☺?
Sodium myristoyl sarcosinate (may be of ANIMAL origin)	Surfactant Antistatic	☺?
Sodium stearate (may be of ANIMAL origin)	Emulsifier Surfactant	☺
Sorbitan palmitate (may be of ANIMAL origin)	Emulsifier	☺
Sorbitan stearate (may be of ANIMAL origin; on the NIH HSDB)	Emulsifier	☺
Spearmint oil (oil of spearmint)	Fragrance Flavoring	☺
Squalane (shark liver oil; of ANIMAL origin)	Lubricant Emollient	☺☺

Potential Effects	Cosmetic Uses	Other Uses
Mucous membrane, eye and skin irritation; dry skin; liver and gastrointestinal toxicity; mouth ulcers; may be toxic to aquatic organisms	Bubble bath, toothpaste, hair conditioner, liquid hand and body wash, body soap, shampoo	Carpet cleaner, dishwashing liquid, pet shampoo
Mild to strong skin irritation; slight eye irritation; slightly toxic to rats in oral doses	Cream shampoo, cleansing cream, bath bombs	
See sarcosines	Foaming face wash	
Non-irritating to the skin; safety is under review	Toothpaste, shaving lather, soap-less shampoo	Chewing gum, animal feeds
Believed safe in cosmetic use; may cause contact dermatitis	Shampoo, hair conditioner, cosmetic cream	
Believed safe in cosmetic use; may cause contact hives	Shampoo, suntan lotion, eyeliner, moisturizer, baby lotion	
Believed to have beneficial health effects; may cause skin rash	Perfume, toothpaste, perfumed cosmetics	Chewing gum, pet shampoo, cigarettes
Believed safe in cosmetic use	Lipstick, shampoo, body wash, moisturizer	

Names	Function	Code	
Stearalkonium chloride (from dimethyl-n-octadecylamine and benzyl chloride; on the NIH HSDB)	Preservative Antistatic agent Emollient	☹	
Stearamide DEA or MEA (may be of ANIMAL origin)	Opacifier Antistatic agent	☹	
Stearyl alcohol (of ANIMAL origin; on the NIH HSDB)	Emollient Opacifier	☺	
Styrene/PVP copolomer (from vinyl pyrrolidone and styrene monomers; styrene is on the NIH HSDB)	Film former Opacifier	☹	
Sulfonamide (sulfanilamide; on the Canadian Hotlist; on the NIH HSDB)	Antibiotic	☹	
Talc and talcum powder (naturally occurring mineral; on the NIH HSDB)	Anti-caking agent Absorbent	☹	
TEA lauryl sulfate (on the NIH HSDB)	Surfactant	☹	

Potential Effects	Cosmetic Uses	Other Uses
Mild skin irritation; severe eye irritation; moderately toxic by ingestion; dermatitis; see quaternary ammonium compounds	Hair conditioner, hair color, lipstick, hair spray	Contraceptive formulations, industrial cleaners
DEA-related ingredient; see diethanolamine	Shampoo, hair conditioner	
May cause allergic reactions and contact dermatitis in people with sensitive skin	Hair conditioner, hair rinse, deodorant, baby lotion, moisturizer, shampoo, eye cream	Pharmaceuticals
See polyvinylpyrrolidone and styrene in section 1	Permanent hair color, liquid eyeliner, cuticle remover	
Itching; skin rash; swelling; hives; kidney toxicity; suspected teratogen	Cosmetics, nail polish	Antibiotic to treat bacterial and fungal infections
Lung irritation; pneumonia; cough; vomiting; ovarian and lung cancer; suspected carcinogen	Face cream, bath powder, baby powder, eye shadow, deodorant, antiperspirant, makeup	
See triethanolamine and sodium lauryl sulfate	Shampoo, bubble bath	Pet shampoo, household cleaners

Names	Function	Code	
Tetrabromofluorescein (synthetic)	Colorant	☹	
Thimerosal (mercury; on the Canadian Hotlist)	Preservative	☹☹	
Thiourea (made by heating a derivative of ammonium cyanide; on the Canadian Hotlist; on the NIH HSDB)	Preservative Additive		
Toluene (derived from petroleum or by distilling Tolu balsam, a plant extract; on the NIH HSDB)	Solvent	☹☹	
Trichloroethane (methyl chloroform)	Solvent Degreaser	☹☹	

Potential Effects	Cosmetic Uses	Other Uses
Photosensitivity; inflammation of lips; respiratory and gastrointestinal symptoms	Indelible lipstick, nail polish	Dyeing of wool, silk and paper
Allergic reactions; contact dermatitis; see mercury compounds	Eye preparations	Filler in vaccines
Allergic reactions: skin irritation; cardiovascular, reproductive and immunotoxicity; recognized carcinogen; toxic to aquatic organisms	Hair dye, hair products, cosmetics	Photography, dye, wet suits, silver polish
Cardiovascular, respiratory, developmental, kidney, liver, reproductive, immuno and neurotoxicity; eye and skin irritation; decreased learning ability; brain damage; toxic to aquatic organisms	Hair gel, perfume, nail polish, hair dye, hairspray	Removing odors in cheese, metal cleaner, adhesive
Cardiovascular, liver, gastrointestinal and neurotoxicity; severe eye and mucous membrane irritation; cardiac arrest; suspected teratogen; toxic to aquatic organisms	Cosmetics, nail polish	Correction fluid, degreaser, glue, spot remover, pre-wash laundry detergent

Names	Function	Code
Triclocarban (prepared from an aniline compound; on the NIH HSDB)	Preservative Antibacterial agent	☹
Triclosan (may contain toxic chemicals; on the Canadian Hotlist; on the NIH HSDB)	Preservative	☹
Triethanolamine (TEA; on the NIH HSDB)	Buffer Coating additive	☹
Zinc oxide (may contain Nanoparticles, see glossary)	Opacifier Additive Colorant	☺?
Zinc stearate (may be of ANIMAL origin)	Colorant	☺?
Zirconium (banned in aerosol cosmetic products; on the Canadian Hotlist; on the NIH HSDB)	Solvent Abrasive	☺?

Potential Effects	Cosmetic Uses	Other Uses
Photoallergic reactions; convulsions; prolonged use may lead to cancer	Deodorant soaps, skin cleansers, medicated cosmetics	Disinfectants, plastics
Toxic if ingested; allergic reactions; contact dermatitis; may be harmful in the environment	Antiperspirant, liquid hand soap, toothpaste, deodorant soap, skin cleanser, mouthwash	Pet shampoo, drugs, detergents, plastic products including toys
Allergic contact dermatitis; skin irritation; may react with nitrites to form nitrosamines	Hand and body lotion, hair conditioner, shave gel, mascara, shampoo	Coating on fresh fruit & vegetables, cream cleanser
Helps protect against UV radiation; may be unsuitable for dry skin; respiratory toxicity; may cause skin eruptions; suspected teratogen	Baby powder, shaving cream, antiperspirant, sunscreen, hair care products, calamine lotion	Used medically as an antiseptic, astringent and protective in skin diseases
Skin and eye irritation; lung problems and pneumonitis	Baby powder, hand cream, face powder	Tablet manufacture
Believed safe in non-aerosol products; toxic by inhalation; respiratory toxicity; contact allergy	Cosmetic cream, antiperspirant, deodorant	Preparation of dyes

GENETIC ENGINEERING
FLYING PIGS AND SUICIDE SEEDS

Genetic engineering (GE), otherwise known as genetic modification (GM), has had enough exposure in the media over the last few years to ensure that most of us have at least heard of it, even if we have a limited understanding of what it is and the implications of its use. Familiar terms such as "frankenfoods" have been coined and used by those opposed to the introduction and spread of this biotechnology. The terms "terminator genes" and "suicide seeds" are less well known. We will briefly look at these later.

First, what does this term genetic engineering actually mean? In its simplest form genetic engineering involves the removal of a particular gene from one species of life and inserting it into another (possibly totally unrelated) life form. Genes are the biological units of heredity, the individual messages that go together to form DNA molecules, the blueprints for the thousands of proteins that combine to form the building blocks of all life from bacteria to humans. Picture it like this book you are reading. The individual letters (genes) are arranged to form words (DNA) that are then assembled to form sentences (proteins) and the sentences link together to eventually become the book (life form). Apart from determining which traits are inherited, genes also control all the activities that take place within the life form over the period of its lifetime. Herein is the reason why pigs cannot fly and birds can. The "flight genes" naturally present in birds are not part of the inherited blueprint of the life form we call a pig.

Since the early 1970s scientists have been able to alter the natural inherited behavior of a life form or organism, by adding genes from another totally unrelated life form. Genes do not work in isolation, but in highly complex relationships that are a long way from being fully understood. Transferring genes between unrelated species can lead to organisms behaving in ways that nature did not intend. (And no, as far as I am aware nobody has yet developed a flying pig.)

Genetic Engineering does not in any way resemble traditional breeding techniques. Traditional breeding techniques operate within established natural boundaries allowing reproduction to take place only between closely related forms. Dairy farmers cross genes from high milk yielding cows with genes from high butterfat yielding cows to produce cows that give lots of milk with high butterfat content. These genes are selected from the "gene pool" of available cow genes. Pigs are bred from a gene pool of available pig genes. However we don't mate cows with pigs. The gene pools remain separate. Different species of tomatoes can cross-pollinate to produce a more frost-hardy species. Always there are natural groupings, with clearly defined boundaries—finely tuned by millions of years of evolution—to work together harmoniously. Genetic engineering, on the other hand, attempts to transfer genes between unrelated species that would never crossbreed in nature. Fish genes are inserted into mice or tomatoes and bacterial genes into maize. One of the concerns of many in the scientific community is that this can give rise to potential health risks. When this biotechnology enters the food chain, the impacts on our health are largely unpredictable. An amino acid supplement that was engineered using GE bacteria caused many deaths and deformities. The Flavr Savr, a tomato genetically modified to increase its shelf life, induced stomach lesions when fed to experimental rats and was later withdrawn from the market. Soybeans engineered with a gene from Brazil nuts caused allergic reactions in people sensitive to nuts. The list of failures goes on.

The fact that natural evolution proceeds at a much slower pace than technology makes this all the more alarming. By unnaturally manipulating our environment and the foods we consume without a true understanding of the consequences, it may be a generation or more before any devastating effects are realized, and probably then too late to reverse them.

Apart from the potential dangers to our health, genetic engineering poses other threats as well. One of the growing industries across the world is a return to organic agriculture. As consumers become more aware of the risks associated with toxic pesticides and herbicides, both to human health and the environment, the demand for chemical-free products increases. Organic food is safer, as organic farming prohibits synthetic pesticide use. Governing bodies have been set up to oversee and regulate this industry. These bodies certify that their members do not use synthetic chemicals in the production of their products. These products comprise foodstuffs, personal care products, cosmetics and the like. Certified organic status also implies freedom from genetically engineered ingredients, additives etc. Farms with certified organic status risk losing this hard-earned status if genetically engineered crops are grown nearby because of the cross-contamination that may occur.

For thousands of years farmers have saved some of the seeds from their crops to plant in the following seasons. This has proved essential to the maintenance and further evolution of agricultural diversity worldwide and is the basis of food security. All this is now in jeopardy with the advent of terminator technology, a marriage between gene technology and nanotechnology. It is officially known as Genetic Use Restriction Technologies (GURTS). Terminator seeds or "suicide seeds" are engineered to be sterile and thereby prevent farmers from saving seed. Scientists use carbon nanofibers to inject synthetic DNA into millions of cells simultaneously.

Some scientists express a concern about what could happen if the terminator is unleashed on the environment. The fear is that terminator technology could migrate from one farm to another or from a farm to wild plants. Questions have been raised like what happens when animals and humans ingest the nanofibres as food? What are the environmental impacts? And where will the nanofibres go when the plant decomposes in the soil? Some see this as an extremely risky and controversial technology. This technology is currently under an international ban. However, if the powerful biotech companies were allowed to introduce it, this would enable corporate monopoly control of global food and fiber production, by preventing seed saving. Since 1998, only public opposition to GURTS has so far curtailed its introduction and only continued public opposition will maintain the ban. Once the ban is lifted, it will be almost impossible to reverse it. And who will benefit from its introduction? Not farmers, not consumers, not the environment. The only winners appear to be a handful of powerful biotech and agribusiness companies.

As yet, GE crops have failed to deliver the promised benefits to farmers and are in fact posing escalating problems for them. GE crops have not been proven safe. On the contrary, sufficient evidence has emerged to give rise to serious safety concerns which, if ignored, could result in irreversible damage to human and animal health and the environment. GE crops pose a continuing threat to non-GE and organic agriculture. Sustainable agriculture, on the other, hand poses none of the threats associated with GE. Research shows that sustainable agriculture results in higher productivity and yields especially in the Developing World. Continued practice results in better-quality soils, a reduction in soil erosion, and a cleaner and safer environment with a reduction in pesticide use without a subsequent increase in pests. Sustainable agriculture leads to healthier and tastier foods with higher nutritional values. Anyone who has eaten homegrown strawberries and other produce, grown without the use of artificial chemicals, will attest to this.

Once released, genetically engineered organisms become part of our ecosystem. Unlike some forms of pollution which may be contained or which may decrease over time, any mistakes we make now will be passed on to all future generations of life. With governments following their own agendas and capitulating to corporate interests, it is up to us to act.

APPENDIX

Safe and/or Beneficial Ingredients Used in Cosmetics and Personal Care Products

Listed below is a small selection of some of the safe and/or beneficial ingredients to look for when shopping for personal care products and cosmetics. It is wise to select products with organic (preferably "certified organic") ingredients, and avoid those with too many synthetic chemicals, especially ones with this ⊗ or this ⊗⊗ symbol. If the product is not certified organic, check the label for evidence that the ingredients are GE-free.

Name	Function
Aloe Vera	botanical
Avocado Oil	natural emollient
Ascorbic Acid (vitamin C)	natural preservative
Candelilla Wax	natural emulsifier
D-Alpha Tocopherol Acetate (vitamin E)	natural preservative
Evening Primrose Oil	botanical
Grapefruit Seed Extract	natural preservative
Hemp Oil	botanical
Honeysuckle Extract	natural fragrance
Jojoba Butter natural	emollient
Jojoba Oil natural	emulsifier
Lecithin (GM-free vegetable origin)	natural humectant
Macadamia Oil natural	emollient
Olive Oil (Castile) Soap	natural surfactant
Panthenol, Dexpanthenol (vitamin B5)	natural emollient

Name	Function
Purified Water natural	solvent
Quince Seed natural	emulsifier
Rice Bran natural	emulsifier
Rosehip Seed Oil natural	emollient
Rosemary Extract natural	preservative
Rose Water natural	perfume
Saffron natural	coloring
Sclerotium Gum	natural emulsifier
Shea Butter natural	emollient
Soapwort	natural surfactant
Stevia	natural sweetener
Vitamin A Palmitate	natural preservative
Xanthan Gum (GE-free)	natural emulsifier
Yucca Extract	natural surfactant

GLOSSARY

abrasive: A substance added to cosmetic products either to remove materials from various body surfaces or to aid mechanical tooth cleaning and improve gloss.

absorbent: A substance added to cosmetic products to take up water and/or oil-soluble dissolved or finely dispersed substances.

acetylated: An organic compound that has had its water removed by heating with acetic anhydride or acetyl chloride. Both these chemicals are hazardous.

additive: A substance added to cosmetic products, often in relatively small amounts, to impart or improve desirable properties or minimize undesirable properties.

allergen: Any substance capable of provoking an inappropriate immune response in susceptible people, but not normally in others.

allergic contact dermatitis: A skin rash caused by direct contact with a substance to which the skin is sensitive. Symptoms may occur anywhere from seven days to many years after repeated low-level exposures, as occurs with cosmetics and personal care products.

allergic reaction: An adverse immune system response involving unusual sensitivity to the action of various environmental stimuli. These stimuli do not normally cause symptoms in the majority of the population.

amines: A class of organic compounds derived from ammonia.

anaphylaxis: Increased sensitivity to the action of an allergen. Symptoms include skin rash, swelling, breathing difficulties and collapse. May cause severe or even fatal shock.

anticaking agent: A substance used in granular foods like salt or flour to assist free flowing.

anticorrosive: Chemicals added to cosmetics to prevent corrosion of the packaging or the machinery used in the manufacture of the cosmetic.

antifoaming agent: A substance added to foods or cosmetics to prevent excessive frothing or foaming, reduce the formation of scum or prevent boiling over during manufacture.

antimicrobial: A substance added to a cosmetic product to help reduce the activities of microorganisms on the skin or body.

antioxidant: A substance added to foods or cosmetics to prevent changes or spoiling due to exposure to air. May be natural or synthetic.

antistatic: A substance used to reduce static electricity by neutralizing electrical charge on a surface.

azo dye: A very large class of dyes made from diazonium compounds and phenol. Many azo dyes are thought to be carcinogenic when used in foods.

binder: A substance added to a solid cosmetic mixture to provide cohesion.

biological additive: A substance, derived from a biological origin, added to a cosmetic product to achieve a specific formulation feature.

bleaching agent: A substance used to artificially bleach and whiten flour. A substance used in a cosmetic product to lighten the shade of hair or skin.

botanical: A substance, derived from plants, added to a cosmetic product to achieve a specific formulation feature.

buffer: A substance added to a food or cosmetic product to adjust, maintain or stabilize the acid/alkali (pH) balance.

Canadian Hotlist: Information about cosmetic ingredients that have the potential for adverse effects or which have been restricted or banned in Canada.

carcinogen: A cancer-causing substance. IARC and NTP list carcinogens in 3 categories. 1 = *confirmed* human carcinogen; 2 = *probable* human carcinogen; 3 = *possible* human carcinogen.

carcinogenic: A substance that is capable of causing cancer.

cardiovascular/blood toxicity: Adverse effects on the cardio-vascular or hematopoietic systems that result from exposure to chemical substances. Exposure can contribute to a variety of diseases; including elevated blood pressure (hypertension), hardening of the arteries (arteriosclerosis), abnormal heartbeat, (cardiac arrhythmia) and decreased blood flow to the heart (coronary ischaemia). Exposure can also reduce the oxygen carrying capacity of red blood cells, disrupt important immunological processes carried out by white blood cells, and induce cancer.

chelating agent: A substance added to a food or cosmetic product to react and form complexes with metal ions that could affect stability and/or appearance.

CIR Expert Panel: A body set up in 1976 by the Cosmetic, Toiletry and Fragrance Association (CTFA) to review the safety of ingredients used in cosmetics.

clarifying agent: A substance that removes small amounts of suspended particles from liquids.

CNS: Central Nervous System—our body's major communication network.

coal tar dye: Dyes that were once made from coal tar but are now commercially produced by a synthetic process. These dyes are extremely complex chemical compounds, which have had inadequate independent testing and often contain toxic impurities.

contact dermatitis: *See allergic contact dermatitis.*

cosmetic acne: Acne caused by applying cosmetics to the skin.

cytotoxin: A substance that is poisonous to cells.

denaturant: A poisonous or unpleasant substance added to alcoholic cosmetics to prevent them being ingested. It is also a substance that changes the natural qualities or characteristics of other substances.

dentifrices: Pastes, powders or liquids for cleaning the teeth.

depilatory: A substance or agent used to remove unwanted body hair.

dermatitis: Inflammation of the skin with pain, redness, burning or itching and fluid build-up.

developmental toxicity: Adverse effects on the developing fetus that result from exposure to chemical substances. Developmental toxicants, sometimes called teratogens, include agents that induce structural malformations and other birth defects, low birth weight, metabolic or biological dysfunction, and psychological or behavioral deficits that become manifest as the child grows.

diluent: A substance used to dilute or dissolve other additives.

DPIM: "Dangerous Properties of Industrial Materials." Ed. Sax & Lewis.

eczema: Wet or dry inflammation of the skin causing redness, pain, itching, scaling, peeling, blistering etc.

EDF: Environmental Defense; provides information on chemicals.

emollient: A substance used to soften and soothe the skin.

emulsifier: A substance used in food or cosmetic products to stabilize mixtures and ensure consistency.

emulsion stabilizer: A substance added to a cosmetic product to help the process of emulsification and to improve formulation stability and shelf life.

endocrine toxicity: Adverse effects on the structure and/or functioning of the endocrine system that result from exposure to chemical substances. The endocrine system is composed of many organs and glands that secrete hormones directly into the bloodstream including the pituitary, hypothalamus, thyroid, adrenals, pancreas, thymus, ovaries and testes. Compounds that are toxic to the endocrine system may cause diseases such as hypothyroidism, diabetes mellitus, hypoglycemia, reproductive disorders and cancer.

EPA: Environmental Protection Agency

ester: A compound formed when an acid reacts with an alcohol by the elimination of water.

ethoxylation: The addition of ethyl (from the gas ethane) and oxygen to a degreasing agent to make it less abrasive and cause it to foam more.

FDA: Food and Drug Administration (USA). It is part of the Public Health Service of the US Department of Health and Human Services.

film former: A substance added to a cosmetic product to produce, when applied, a continuous film on skin hair or nails.

flavor enhancer: Chemicals that enhance the taste or odor of food without contributing any taste or odor of their own.

flavoring: The largest category of food additives. Over two thousand synthetic and natural flavorings added to foods to impart the desired flavor.

fragrance: Any natural or synthetic substance used to impart an odor to a product.

fungicide: A substance used to kill or inhibit the growth of fungi.

gelling agent: A substance that is capable of forming a jelly.

GM: Abbreviation for Genetically Modified.

GMO: Genetically Modified Organism.

glazing agent: A substance used to provide a shiny appearance or a protective coat to a food.

GRAS: Generally Recognized As Safe. A list, established by the U.S. Congress in 1958, of substances added to food over a long time.

hazardous chemical agents: 1. Those chemical agents known to have undesirable biological effects, either acutely or chronically, reasonable regard being given to the size of the dose, duration and type of exposure, and the physical state of the compound required to produce such effects. 2. Those agents for which toxicity information is not available, but are highly suspect for reasons of similarity in chemical structure or function to known toxic agents. 3. Those agents that are explosive or violently reactive.

herbicide: A substance used to kill or inhibit the growth of unwanted plants.

hives: An allergic disorder marked by raised, fluid-filled patches of skin or mucous membrane, usually accompanied by intense itching. Also known as nettle rash and urticaria.

HSBD: Hazardous Substances Databank. A data bank of potentially hazardous chemicals found in cosmetics and household products.

humectant: A substance used to hold and retain moisture to prevent a food or product from drying out.

hydrogenated: Liquid oils in food and cosmetic products are converted to semisolid fats at room temperature by adding hydrogen under high pressure. Hydrogenated fats and oils contribute to cancer, heart disease and atheroma.

hydrolysed Turned partly into water as a result of a chemical process.

immunotoxicity: Adverse effects on the functioning of the immune system that result from exposure to chemical substances. Altered immune function may lead to the increased incidence or severity of infectious diseases or cancer, since the immune system's ability to respond adequately to invading agents is suppressed. Toxic agents can also cause autoimmune diseases, in which healthy tissue is attacked by an immune system that fails to differentiate self-antigens from foreign antigens.

intermediate: A chemical substance found as part of a necessary step between one organic compound and another.

kidney toxicity: Adverse effects on the kidney, ureter or bladder that result from exposure to chemical substances. Some toxic agents cause acute injury to the kidney, while others produce chronic changes that can lead to end stage renal failure or cancer. The consequences of renal failure can be profound, sometimes resulting in permanent damage that requires dialysis or kidney transplantation.

liver/gastrointestinal toxicity: Adverse effects on the structure and/or functioning of the gastrointestinal tract, liver, or gall bladder that result from exposure to chemical substances. The liver is frequently subject to injury induced by chemicals, called hepatotoxins, because of its role as the body's principal site of metabolism.

material safety data sheets (MSDS): Data compiled by manufacturers of chemicals providing information on health hazards and safe handling procedures.

miliaria: Acute itchy skin condition occurring as an eruption of spots or blisters resembling millet seeds.

modifier: A substance that induces or stabilizes particular shades in hair colorants.

musculoskeletal toxicity: Adverse effects on the structure and/or functioning of the muscles, bones and joints that result from exposure to chemical substances. Exposure to toxic substances such as coal dust and cadmium has been shown to cause adverse changes to the musculoskeletal system. The bone disorders arthritis, fluorosis and osteomalacia are among the musculoskeletal diseases that can be induced by occupational or environmental toxicants.

mutagen: Any substance that induces mutation or permanent changes to genetic material (DNA) of cells.

mutagenic: Capable of causing mutations. Can be induced by stimuli such as certain food chemicals, pesticides and radiation.

nanoparticles: Anything smaller than 100 nanometers (a nanometer is a billionth of a meter) in size or more than 800 times smaller than a human hair. They can enter the bloodstream and cross the blood-brain barrier.

necrosis: Cell death.

neurotoxicity: Adverse effects on the structure or functioning of the central and/or peripheral nervous system that result from exposure to chemical substances. Symptoms of neurotoxicity include muscle weakness, loss of sensation and motor control, tremors, alterations in cognition, and impaired functioning of the autonomic nervous system.

NIH: National Institutes of Health.

NIOSH: The National Institute of Occupational Safety and Health, which is the research arm of the US Occupational Safety and Health Administration (OSHA).

nitrosamines: Potential carcinogenic compounds formed when an amine reacts with a nitrosating agent or substances containing nitrites.

nitrosating agent: A substance capable of introducing nitrogen and oxygen molecules into a compound that may cause the compound to form potential carcinogenic nitrosamines.

NRC: Not recommended for young children and infants.

NTP: National Toxicology Program (USA). Provides information on chemical toxicity.

opacifier: A substance added to a shampoo or other transparent or translucent liquid cosmetic product to make it impervious to visible light or nearby radiation.

oral care agent: A substance added to a personal care product for the care of the oral cavity.

oxidising agent: A substance added to a food or cosmetic product to change the chemical nature of another substance by adding oxygen.

photoallergy: *See photosensitivity.*

photosensitivity: A condition in which the application to the body or ingestion of certain chemicals causes skin problems (rash, pigmentation changes, swelling etc) when the skin is exposed to sunlight.

phototoxicity: Reaction to sunlight or ultraviolet light resulting in inflammation.

plasticizer: A substance added to impart flexibility and workability without changing the nature of a material.

preservative: A substance added to food and cosmetic products to inhibit the growth of bacteria, fungi and viruses.

propellant: A gas used to expel the contents of containers in the form of aerosols.

reagent: A substance used for the detection of another substance by chemical or microscopic means.

reducing agent: A substance added to food and cosmetic products to decrease, deoxidize or concentrate the volume of another substance.

reproductive toxicity: Adverse effects on the male and female reproductive systems that result from exposure to chemical substances. Reproductive toxicity may be expressed as alterations in sexual behavior, decreases in fertility or loss of the fetus during pregnancy. A reproductive toxicant may interfere with the sexual functioning or reproductive ability of exposed individuals from puberty throughout adulthood.

respiratory toxicity: Adverse effects on the structure or functioning of the respiratory system that result from exposure to chemical substances. The respiratory system consists of the nasal passages, pharynx, trachea, bronchi and lungs. Respiratory toxicants can produce a variety of acute and chronic pulmonary conditions, including local irritation, bronchitis, pulmonary edema, emphysema and cancer.

RTECS: The Registry of Toxic Effects of Chemical Substances.

sensitization: Heightened immune response following repeated contact with an allergen.

sequestrant: A substance capable of attaching itself to unwanted trace metals such as cadmium, iron and copper that cause deterioration in food and cosmetic products by advancing the oxidation process.

solvent: A substance added to food and cosmetic products to dissolve or disperse other components.

stabilizer: A substance added to a product to give it body and to maintain a desired texture.

surface active agent: A substance that reduces surface tension when dissolved in solution. These agents fall into three categories: detergents, wetting agents, and emulsifiers.

surfactant: A wetting agent that lowers the surface tension of a liquid substance, allowing it to spread out and penetrate more easily. Surfactants fall into four main categories: anionic, non-ionic, cationic, and amphoteric.

tenderizer: A substance or process used to alter the structure of meat to make it less tough and more palatable.

teratogen: *See developmental toxicity.*

teratogenic: Capable of causing defects in a developing fetus.

texturizer: A substance used to improve the texture of various foods or cosmetics.

thickener: A substance used to add viscosity and body to foods, lotion and cream.

UV absorber: A substance added to a cosmetic product to filter ultra-violet (UV) rays so as to protect the skin or the product from the harmful effects of these rays.

viscosity controlling agent: A substance added to a cosmetic product to increase or decrease the viscosity (flowability) of the finished product.

xenoestrogen: An environmental compound that has estrogen-like activity thereby mimicking the properties of the hormone estrogen.

USEFUL INTERNET RESOURCES

The following links to Internet websites have been included here to give you a starting place for doing your own research. All links were accessible at the time of writing.

American Association of Allergy, Asthma and Immunology	www.aaaai.org
Canadian Celiac Association	www.celiac.ca
Cancer Prevention Coalition	www.preventcancer.com
Center for Science in the Public Interest	www.cspinet.org
Environmental Defense Fund	www.edf.org
Environmental Working Group	www.ewg.org
Food Allergy and Anaphylaxis Network	www.foodallergy.org
Food and Behavior Research	www.fabresearch.org
International Agency for Research on Cancer (IARC)	www.iarc.fr
Leading Edge International Research Group	www.truefax.org
Material Safety Data Sheets	www.msdssearch.com
National Toxicology Program	http://ntp.niehs.nih.gov
National Library of Medicine	www.ncbi.nlm.nih.gov/pubmed
Organic Consumers Association	www.organicconsumers.org

BIBLIOGRAPHY

Agency for Toxic Substances and Disease Registry, (ATSDR)

American Academy of Dermatology

Antczak, Dr. Stephen and Gina, "Cosmetics Unmasked," *Thorsons*, 2001

Australian Consumers Association

Cancer Prevention Coalition

Center for Science in the Public Interest (CSPI)

Commonwealth Scientific and Industrial Research Organisation (CSIRO), Australia

Crumpler, Diane, "Chemical Crisis," *Scribe Publications*

Cummins, Ronnie and Ben Lilliston, *Genetically Engineered Food—A Self Defense Guide for Consumers*, second edition, Marlow & Company, 2004

Day, Phillip, "Cancer—Why We're Still Dying to Know the Truth," *Credence Publications*, 2000

Day, Phillip, "Health Wars," *Credence Publications*, 2001

Department of Food Science and Technology (UK)

Dingle, Peter and Toni Brown, "Dangerous Beauty—Cosmetics and Personal Care," *Healthy Home Solution*, 1999

Epstein, Samuel S. M.D., "Unreasonable Risk," *Environmental Toxicology*, 2002

Environmental Defense

Environmental Protection Agency (EPA), (USA)

Environmental Working Group

Food and Drug Administration (FDA), (USA)

Food Standards Agency (UK)

Food Standards Australia New Zealand, (FSANZ)

Hampton, Aubrey, *What's in Your Cosmetics*, Organica Press

Hanssen, Maurice, with Jill Marsden, *The New Additive Code Breaker*, Lothian, 1991

In-Tele-Health, Hyperhealth Natural Health & Nutrition CD-ROM, 2005 Ed.

International Agency for Research on Cancer (IARC)

Joint Expert Committee on Food Additives (JECFA)

Journal of the American Medical Association (JAMA)

Journal of the American College of Toxicology

Lancet, The Leading Edge Research

Material Safety Data Sheets (MSDS), from numerous sources

National Center for Environmental Health

National Food Safety Database

National Institutes of Health (NIH), (USA)

National Institute of Occupational Safety and Health (NIOSH)

National Libraries of Medicine (USA)

National Resources Defense Council

National Toxicology Program (USA), (NTC)

Organic Consumers Association

Organic Federation of Australia

Registry of Toxic Effects of Chemical Substances, The, (RTECS)

Sax and Lewis, *Dangerous Properties of Industrial Materials*, Seventh Edition

Sargeant, Doris, and Karen Evans, *Hard to Swallow—The Truth About Food Additives*, Alive Books, 1999

Steinman, David and Samuel S. Epstein, *The Safe Shopper's Bible*, Macmillan, 1995

Taubert, P.M., "Silent Killers," *CompSafe Consultancy*, 2001

Taubert, P.M., "Your Health and Food Additives—2000 Edition," *CompSafe Consultancy*

Taubert, P.M., "Read the Label, Know the Risks," *CompSafe Consultancy*, 2004

Total Environment Centre, *A-Z of Chemicals in the Home*, 4th edition

Winter, Ruth M.S., *A Consumer's Dictionary of Cosmetic Ingredients—Sixth Edition*, Three Rivers Press, 2005

Winter, Ruth M.S., *A Consumer's Dictionary of Food Additives—Sixth Edition*, Three Rivers Press, 2004

ABOUT THE AUTHOR

Bill Statham lives with his wife and business partner Kay Lancashire in Victoria, Australia. He is a researcher, writer, and publisher with an interest in health education, and is committed to making a positive difference to the health of people and the environment.

He studied and practiced homeopathy both in Australia and England for over ten years. During this time he became increasingly concerned about the detrimental effects on people's health caused by synthetic chemicals in the foods we eat and products we use every day.

Bill wrote *What's in Your Food?* (originally titled *The Chemical Maze*) to make it simpler and easier for people to recognize those additives and ingredients in foods, personal care products and cosmetics having the potential to cause discomfort and ill health. With this recognition comes freedom of choice, and for many a new lease of life.